2 Great Diabetic Food Plans in one Cookbook for the newly diagnosed

The Plant and not the Vegetable-Based Diet, Over 100 Delicious and Easy Recipes for diabetics

by Karen Berenice Harper

TABLE OF CONTENTS

INTRODUCTION **5**

CHAPTER 1 .... **7**

1.1. INTRODUCTION ABOUT TYPE-2 DIABETICS 7
1. 11 *What It Means To Be Diagnosed With Type-2 Diabetic* 7
1. 12 *Risk Factors causing Type 2 Diabetics* 10
1. 13. *How to do Testing of Type 2 Diabetics* 11
1. 14 *Preventive Measures to Manage and Control Diabetics* 14
1. 15 *Complications Arising Due to Diabetics* 23
1.2. DIABETIC NUTRITION & HOW TO CHOOSE THE RIGHT FOOD 24
1.21 *Nutritional Basics concerning Diabetics* 25
1.22 *How to Choose the Right Food* 27
1.3. FOOD LABELLING & DIABETICS 29
1. 4. GLYCEMIC INDEX AND CONTROLLING DIABETICS 31

CHAPTER 2 .... **45**

2.1. MEAL PLANNING & DIABETIC MANAGEMENT 45
2.21 *Week Meal Plan for Non-Vegetarians* 46
2.22 *Week Meal Plan for Vegetarians* 61

CHAPTER 3 .... **76**

3.1. BREAKFAST RECIPES 76
3.2 LUNCH 114
3.3 DINNER 154
3.4 SMOOTHIES & JUICES 194
3.5 DESSERTS 234
3.6 EXTRA RECIPES 274

CONCLUSION **322**

INTRODUCTION

Do you love Tom Hanks? If you are an adherent fan of the actor, then you should read the following quote, which is motivational. He says, "I have high blood sugar, and Type 2 diabetics are not going to kill me. But I just to have eat right, and exercise, and lose weight, and watch what I eat, and I will be fine for the rest of my life". And I believe this is the attitude we also need to have in our life when we come face to face with diabetics.

With 100 recipes tailored for individuals with diabetics while being tempting for everyone, this diabetic cookbook is ideal for everyone. The book provides all the information about diabetics along with a customizable 4-week meal plan, which could be particularly helpful for the newly diagnosed. The 4-week clearly defined meal plan offers you the easiest way to manage your type-2 diabetics and your diet. On top, the meal plan is easy to follow. It can avoid all side-effects of misleading foods while aiding in maintaining healthy blood sugar levels.

Furthermore, the book offers not only comprehensive content that features information about Type-2 diabetics but also a multitude of delicious recipes that you will enjoy. There are recipes for diabetic breakfasts, lunch, dinner, green smoothies, and juices. All the recipes in it deliver exceptional flavor and maximum nutrition, which genuinely benefits those battling diabetics. A healthy lifestyle starts in the kitchen.

With the support and guidance of this book, you will be able to thrive with diabetics. I can assure you will like this book because it is informative. What's more, the book contains:

- Two customizable 4-weeks meal plan each for vegetarians and non-vegetarians.
- The book also has complete and updated information on type-2 diabetics and how to control it.
- + 100 diabetic-friendly recipes across all categories & complete nutritional information for all these.

By learning to cook healthy fresh food, you would be able to combat against diabetics effectively. Rather than considering it as a difficult problem to handle, the whole process should be an enjoyable course that could save your life straightforwardly. Therefore, a cookbook with reliable recipes & tons of information is a must-have as you can use it all the time. So why postpone buying this book anymore? Get it now, and live the healthy lifestyle you always dreamed!

CHAPTER 1

1.1. INTRODUCTION ABOUT TYPE-2 DIABETICS

1. 11 What It Means To Be Diagnosed With Type-2 Diabetic

Irrespective of whether you have been on this diabetic journey for a long time or newly diagnosed, there would be times. Times when you would get overwhelmed and confused about how you can lead a healthy diabetic lifestyle. But then, let me tell you that managing and controlling diabetics isn't an issue provided you have the right attitude.

Earlier for the treatment of diabetics, depending on the type of disease, diet therapy, and medication, was given preference. But for the last few years, patient education has been given high priority by WHO, and hence officially included in the therapeutic arsenal of diabetic treatment. An article published in the US PMC by the IRCMJ (https://www.ncbi.nlm.nih.gov/pmc/articles/PMC3964421/) and by other several studies, pointed out that, if at the onset of the disease, the patient is adequately educated about his health condition and taught how to manage it competently, his attitude towards its management would be positive.

Refining the quality of life of the patient so that it becomes closer to the lifestyle of a healthy person is what the medical practitioners are trying to achieve these days. Your diabetic treatment will be adequate if you can reduce the risk of severe hypoglycemia episodes and normalize blood sugar levels.

Therefore, before you start the whole process of managing your diabetics, getting the necessary information about diabetics can be helpful. As you might already know, **type-2 diabetes is a medical condition wherein your body is not able to use insulin the way it should.** Insulin resistance gets observed in these conditions. Earlier, it affected only middle-aged people and the elderly, but then now it is seen even in kids and teens. Childhood obesity is one of the reasons behind this.

Now, what is insulin, and what does it do? Insulin is a hormone formed by the pancreas and is released into the body when the food gets broken down. The hormone turns the sugar you eat from the food into glucose and transport it from the blood to cells for energy. But, when you have diabetics, the cells do not produce a sufficient amount of insulin or are not able to use insulin properly. So when you eat carbohydrates, the glucose that breaks down stays in your blood instead of being transported to the cells where they are supposed to be. This accumulation of blood sugar in your blood is known as high blood sugar.

When the body isn't able to use insulin to bring glucose to the cells, the body relies on other alternatives energy sources in your tissue, muscles, and organs. On top, it also forces the pancreas to work harder to produce more insulin, and the body's cell gets starved for energy. All these cause several chain reactions, which in turn leads to the early symptoms of diabetics gradually.

For a long time, the disease may not manifest itself at all; therefore, the symptoms appear gradually, and people often seek help late. A lot of liquid and salts from the body gets released through the kidneys. Some of the early signs of type 2 diabetics are:

- constant hunger
- being very thirsty
- frequent urination
- loss of energy
- blurry vision
- fatigue
- wounds that won't heal. The symptoms, though, would vary from person to person.

Though diabetics is a long-lasting disease condition, it is different from other chronic diseases as it can be self-managed through proper medication and diet. What you do every day will impact your health in the long-run. So making healthy changes in your diet and lifestyle every day can make a big difference regarding how you handle diabetics. Alongside independent determination of glucose levels regularly is also integral. Therefore, through your active involvement in the treatment, diabetics can be managed.

1. 12 Risk Factors causing Type 2 Diabetics

They are certain factors that make you more susceptible to diabetics. Some of the elements, as mentioned in a study published in the International Journal of Medical Sciences & https://www.ncbi.nlm.nih.gov/pmc/articles/PMC4166864/, are:

- **Genetic predisposition** – Family genes can affect how your body makes insulin. The risk of getting diabetics from genes ranges from 10% if one parent suffers from it to 50% if both the parents are affected by it.
- **Obesity** – Being overweight can cause insulin resistance, especially for the fat accumulated around the waist. More fatty tissues mean a higher chance for the cells to become more resistant to insulin.
- **Broken Beta Cells** – When the cells that make insulin sends the wrong signal, the blood sugar level gets thrown off.
- **Age** – For those aged above 45 years and above, they are more susceptible.

- Having high triglycerides level
- Having heart & heart blood vessel diseases
- **Little exercise or a sedentary lifestyle** – This increases your risk of getting diabetics. Exercise helps the cells to respond better to insulin.
- Bad Sleeping Habits
- Smoking

1. 13. How to do Testing of Type 2 Diabetics

One of the best ways to test for diabetics is through a blood test. We can get a lot of information from blood work. Diagnostic testing for diabetics includes:

- **Haemoglobin A1C Test** – This test measures the level of blood glucose over the past two or three months.
- **Fasting Plasma Glucose** – Also known as fasting blood sugar test, this test is done by measuring blood sugar on an empty stomach.
- **Oral Glucose Tolerant Test** – This test measures the blood glucose level before and after you drink something sweet to understand how your body handles the sugar.

Below is a table showing the expected indicators for the HbAic level glucose for different age groups concerning glycemia and HbA levels.

(The chart gets based on a study done by Petunina NA, Goncharova EV, Terekhova AL. Management of diabetes mellitus. The new period of self-control: detection of Glucose trends and patterns. Diabetes mellitus. 2017;20(6):441-448. doi: 10.14341/DM8254).

Link: Source of the GI table:

Categories of Patients with diabetics	HBA (IC) % Normal Scores	Plasma Glucose on an empty stomach (Before meals)	Plasma Glucose 2 hours after eating
Young age without the risk of severe hypoglycemia	<6.5	<6.5	<8
Young age with risk of severe hypoglycemia & Middle age the risk of severe hypoglycemia	<7	<7	9
Middle age with the risk of severe hypoglycemia & Elderly without the risk of severe hypoglycemia	<7.5	<7.5	<10.0
Elderly with the risk of severe hypoglycemia	<8.0	<8.0	<11.0

Below is a table from the Diabetics Journal site showing an average blood sugar level at different times during the day.

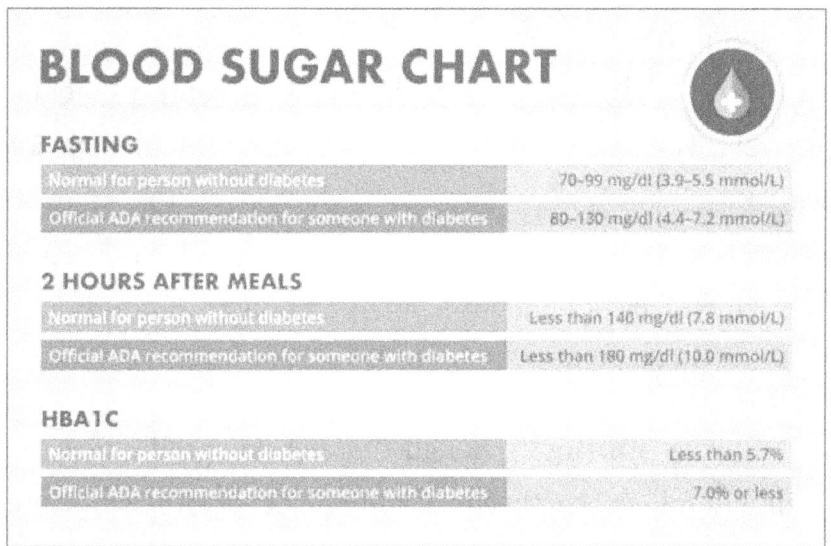

Here is another table from the Diabetescouncil, showing the average blood sugar levels for type 1 and typ2 diabetics patients.

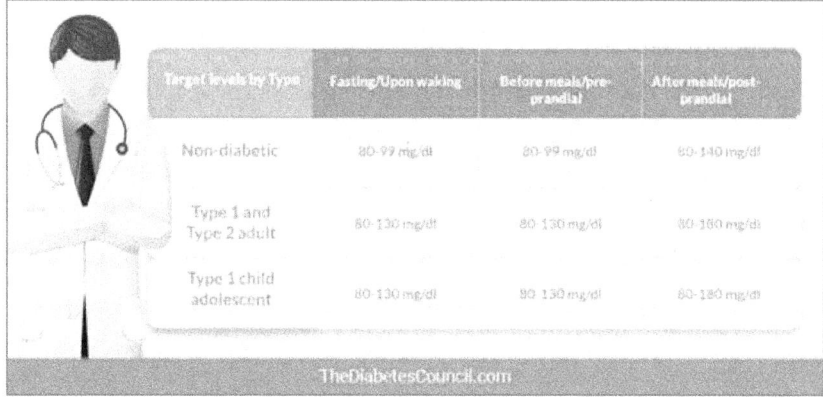

1. 14 Preventive Measures to Manage and Control Diabetics

By adopting healthy changes to your diet and lifestyle along with proper medication, you will be able to control diabetics effectively. The goal should be to stay within a healthy specific range. Based on several reports dedicated to the study of preventive measures against diabetics, to reach your target blood sugar levels and to remain robust, precautionary measures can be taken.

- **Healthy Eating** - Though there is no specific diet that you should follow strictly concerning diabetics, it is sufficient, as long as you eat healthy fresh food. The combination of healthy eating and optimal physical activity can benefit us from avoiding the complications arising from this disease. Just make a note of the below nutritional guidelines before making and consuming each meal.
- **Cut back on refined carbohydrates**, especially sugary drinks, sweets, trans fat, and saturated fats - Going through your diet and making the necessary changes is the primary step towards preventing diabetes. Food ingredients that have sugar and refined carbohydrates in large amounts can cause severe health complications. The sugar molecules formed as a result of this breakdown of carbohydrates stay in the blood.

Studies & prove there is a correlation between the intake of foods high in refined carbohydrates and a rise in the likelihood of the disease. If you reduce having such food, the risk gets diminished. Of the thirty-seven studies done to date, all have confirmed that people who devour fast carbohydrates are 40% more expected to have diabetes.

- **Get adequate fiber in all your meals** - Foods rich in fiber are excellent for health while facilitating to sustain both insulin and sugar at optimal levels. Fiber absorbs liquid and forms a kind of jelly mixture in the digestive tract that decelerates down the processes of digestion and hence slower flow of sugar into the blood. Insoluble fiber also thwarts sugar from rising sharply, but the precise mechanism of action of this substance is not fully known. High fiber foods should be in the diet provided not exposed to much heat treatment.

- **Include a large number of vitamin substances, minerals, and fiber, especially vitamin D** - Cholecalciferol is one of the most vital vitamins directly related to blood sugar control. Lesser the amount of this vitamin in the body, the higher the risks of the disease. The ideal level of its content is measured to be at least 30 ng / ml.

Studies published in the Diabetes Spectrum by ADA have pointed out that owing to the high concentration of vitamin D in the blood, the probability of getting type 2 diabetes is lowered by 55% in adults. In Finland, observing the health of children taking supplements with cholecalciferol exhibited that their risk of developing type 1 diabetes reduced by 78%.

Vitamin D has a positive effect on the cells that synthesize insulin, regularizes sugar, and lessens the likelihood of diabetes. To make up for its daily norm, which is equal to 2000 and up to 4000 ME, being in the sun, eating cod liver, and fatty fish varieties can be an excellent idea.

- **Smaller food portions help** - Eat at regular intervals say 5 to 7 times a day, and this applies to both dietary and conventional nutrition. For those suffering from obesity, the food portions should be small. The more food you consume at a time, the higher your sugar and insulin levels rise. And if you eat food in smaller helpings, you can evade sharp surges. Ensure that you don't skip meals.

A study that showed that the size of food intake affects the likelihood of developing diabetes continued for two years. Experimentally, the risk of getting diabetes was lowered by 46% after swapping from gigantic portions to small ones. Another experiment substantiated that thanks to small servings, you can notice a difference in the state of both insulin and blood levels after three months.

- **Lessen the amount of heat-treatment of food** – The cooking technique employed while cooking affects a person's health directly. Additional preservatives and vegetable oils used in cooking have an undesirable impact on increasing the incidence of diabetes. Plant-based foods, vegetables, nuts, and fruits, i.e., wholesome foods, avert these risks. The foremost thing to take note is that there is less exposure to thermal effects. Ready-made products surge the likelihood of disease by 30%, and "raw products," on the contrary, lowers it.

- **Consuming tea and coffee** - Along with water, you should include coffee and tea in your daily diet. A study published by Diabetologia points that having coffee/tea consumption at least three times a day can decrease the risk of diabetes by 42%. Tea has a comparable effect, specifically on overweight people and women.

Tea and coffee encompass antioxidants called polyphenols. They attack diabetes while defending the body from this disease. Another antioxidant component, but present only in green tea, is EGCG or epigallocatechin gallate, which reduces sugar and raises the body's susceptibility to insulin.

- **Include curcumin and berberine in your diet** - Curcumin is one of the components of turmeric, a spice that is the foundation of curry. It has powerful anti-inflammatory properties and gets used in Ayurveda generously. The substance impeccably aids in coping with arthritis and has a positive effect on many markers accountable for diabetes.

In the study, which lasted nine months, was attended by 240 people. All of them were in the risk group; that is, they had a predisposition to diabetes. The entire experiment participants took 750 mg of the substance per day; as a result, all had zero progression of chronic disease. Besides, each participant improved their degree of insulin sensitivity, enhanced the function of cells responsible for the production of this hormone.

Berberine - It is a part of herbs traditionally used in Chinese folk medicine for several millennia. Like curcumin, this herb also lessens inflammatory processes and helps to get clear of harmful cholesterol.

There are about fourteen scientific readings that have established the fact that berberine has properties similar to Metformin — the most famed of the ancient drugs for the treatment of diabetes and in lowering sugar. Nevertheless, no direct studies to test the effects of the matter on people who are at risk took place. However, if you decide to take berberine, you should first check with the doctor, since it is quite strong.

- **Proper Exercise** – If possible, try to get half to one hour of physical and aerobic exercise every day. Any workout that raises your heart rate would be perfect for keeping your heart healthy and for controlling blood sugar. Furthermore, physical activity can intensify the sensitivity of cells to insulin, which in turn permits the pancreas not to yield this hormone in massive amounts. Accordingly, it becomes much easier for the body to sustain sugar levels. For example, brisk walking for thirty minutes is an excellent idea as it can cut the risk by 30%.

And if it is light exercise, five times a week, it lowers the risk of type II diabetes by 50%.

Scientists have found that high — intensity exercises escalate the body's sensitivity to insulin by 85%, and moderately by 51%. The effect, though, can be seen only on those days you do the exercise. The result happens as the outcome of strength, high-intensity, and aerobic training. If you make physical exercise a slice of your life, then insulin will begin to be formed without any disorders. To make this easier to attain, you should select the type of activity that you prefer the most so that you won't miss even one day.

- **Reducing weight among obese people** - Diabetes tends to affects people with excess body weight. If there is an increased risk of getting the disease, then the fat accumulated around the liver and abdominal cavity is the most responsible for it. The excess becomes the key reason that the body becomes less sensitive to insulin, which surges the risk of diabetes.

Given this fact, even minute weight loss is a reason for noteworthy improvements and can bring about prevention of the disease. The more weight lost, the better. In one experiment with about a thousand participants, losing weight per kilogram reduced the risk of developing the disease by 16%. The maximum attainment during the study was a remarkable 96%.

To lose excess body weight, you should follow a diet. It can be Mediterranean, vegetarian, or any food plan that does not damage your health. It is imperative not only to reduce weight but also to keep up the achieved result. Along with the returning kilograms, old difficulties will come up again with more intensity.

- **Observation of blood sugar levels regularly** – Checking the concentration of sugar in the body at regular intervals can assist in the better management of diabetics. Monitoring your pressure and glucose levels on your own between doctor visits is essential.
- **Avoid sedentary lifestyle** - Absence of movement plays a vital role in the development of the disease, according to scientists involved in the study of diabetics. There were 47 different studies conducted, and in all of them, there was a link between a sedentary lifestyle and a 91% increase in risk factors. To avoid a sedentary lifestyle, set realistic, achievable goals. Getting up every hour from the table and walking around the office, taking the staircase instead of the elevator, or talking on the phone standing, rather than sitting, are all relatively easy targets.
- **Intake of medications or insulin on time** is also essential to maintain average blood sugar levels.
- **Consume more water** – Drink more water rather than depending on juices, sugary juices, and carbonated drinks. These drinks comprise sugar, preservatives, and other

additives that are not always recognized by the consumer. According to a recent study, consuming carbonated drinks escalates the likelihood of developing LADA, that is, type 1 diabetes, which upsets people aged 18 and older. The most extensive study on this aspect encompassed about 2,800 persons. In persons who had two bottles of carbonated sweet juices a day, the risk of developing type 2 diabetes increased by 20, and type 1 diabetes increased by 99 percent. Fruit juices can also be a factor.

Water satiates your thirst and can control your insulin sugar levels. This effect was found in an experiment when a group of people suffering from overweight, was given ordinary water instead of soda. All participants had not only lowered sugar levels but also increased their sensitivity to insulin.

- **Trying out the low-carb diet** – The ketogenic diet, a low carb diet is one of the most effective diets for those who want to lose weight without much harm. The food plan is suggested as a precautionary measure, both because of its excellent results in losing pounds while decreasing insulin resistance.

During a three-month experiment, half of the people followed a low-carb diet, and the other half a low-fat one. The low-carb plan people showed a reduction in sugar concentration by 12% and insulin-by 50% compared to those who took a low-fat diet. Pointers of the second group were much more modest and accounted for only 1% of the drop in sugar and 19% in insulin. This best validates the benefits of a low-carb diet. An artificially created carbohydrate deficit permits you to keep sugar before and after meals almost the same. Thus, the pancreas will not produce a large amount of insulin, which is a deterrence to diabetes.

There is another study for people prone to diabetes, which pointed out that due to the ketogenic diet, blood sugar fell to 92 mmol / l, that is, it fell to the norm, although it was at 118 before.

- **Normalization of psycho-emotional state** – Stress, and anxiety can lead to metabolic diseases like obesity and the development of diabetics. For that matter, it is essential for stress resistance to be reliable.
- **Create a diabetic action plan for health emergencies** - When you feel unwell because of other medical conditions, your sugar levels elevates. During these times, stress hormones apply their effects on the liver and cause the liver to release more glucose. Increased levels, in turn, makes the work of the body more complicated.

High levels of glucose in the blood can result in dehydration, and at times can be even life-threatening. So to avoid all that, it is always better to consult your doctor and create a diabetics management action plan for emergency health situations based on your medical history.

1. 15 Complications Arising Due to Diabetics

Type-2 diabetics, do not pose a direct threat to a person's life. But then, if unmanaged, the disease can slowly progress that can harmfully affect the functionality of all the internal organs and body systems. The likelihood of getting cardiovascular system is quite significant for those who suffer from type-2 diabetics. Some of the other main complications that can arise are:

- **Diabetic Microangiopathy** – In this, the vascular walls of the blood vessels, especially that of the small get affected adversely.
- **Polyneuropathy** – The central nervous system gets affected by this.
- Renal or Kidney Failure
- **Eye Diseases** like glaucoma and cataracts
- **Severe Joint Pain** – Diabetics can also affect the musculoskeletal system, which in turn can lead to severe joint pain.

1.2. DIABETIC NUTRITION & HOW TO CHOOSE THE RIGHT FOOD

As Hippocrates said, "Let your food be your medicine." Along with proper medication and exercise, food plays a vital role in controlling diabetics. Adequate nutrition is the stepping stone of effective treatment. When your meals are healthy, they aid you in achieving a healthier weight and to maintain a steady level of blood sugar levels. A healthy diet reduces your risk of further health complications. Whatever be the diet or food plan you follow, make sure it meets your body needs.

Once diagnosed with diabetics, it doesn't mean that you should abandon all your favorite foods. Similarly, you should never go for a strict diet and try to lose weight instantly. Rather than concentrating merely on what foods you shouldn't eat and what you should, it is always better to look at the whole meal plan or the complete picture. Get a proper idea regarding what you need to do to be healthy rather than picking on minute details.

Always know what you are eating rather than what you are avoiding. Elimination or avoidance can't alone make you healthy. Look at all the food ingredients that you can add to increase your immunity power and to nourish yourselves. That's what diabetic food-management should be. A whole-diet technique that focuses on all types of nutrients rather than calories is the one you should follow. Every time you take a meal, take more than half an amount of non-starchy carbohydrates, a quarter amount of healthy protein, and fats. And you would be good to go.

1.21 Nutritional Basics concerning Diabetics

A healthy diet is essential to keep your blood glucose levels within safe and healthy levels. But then, the food for diabetic patients is the same as it is for ordinary people. Few points to be noted are:

- Eat meals and snacks on time and at regular intervals. If possible, eat often say 5 to 7 times a day. Similarly, eat food at the same time.
- To consume foods that are nutrient-dense and low in empty calories.
- Avoid or limit the use of salt and alcohol.
- Portion control - When you overeat, it leads to weight gain. So to avoid that, you can eat high-fiber foods, as they can make you feel satiated for a longer time, which in turn can help to portion control.
- Read food labels carefully to understand hidden carbohydrates. For example, avoid foods that have the word 'hydrogenated' in it. They could potentially have trans-fat, which is bad for diabetics.

Along with the above points, ensure that you include the following groups of macronutrients into your meals daily. Macronutrients play an essential role in the proper maintenance and growth of your body. They are:

- **Carbohydrates** – Carbs are an integral source of energy for the optimal working of the body. Rather than eliminating them from your diet, you should try to include them based on the type of carbohydrates. Complex carbohydrates and simple sugar are the two main divisions here. Starches and fiber take more time to digest as they are complex. Simple sugar, on the other hand, has the potential to raise sugar levels quickly because they absorb readily. Be mindful of the rate and the amount you consume rather than complete elimination.

- **Proteins** -Protein can give a steady amount of energy with little effect on blood sugar. On top, they can keep your feeling full for a more extended time. For this reason, you can always include them in your daily meals. They are two types of protein; plant-based protein and animal-based protein. Include both kinds of protein in equal amounts. Protein-packed foods include eggs, dairy, legumes, and forth on.

- **Fat** – Fat takes a longer time to digest and can keep you feel for a longer time. They perform several useful functions for the body and is an essential component of the diet. Healthy fats should be integral to your diet. Alongside, fat is a concentrated fuel source, providing more amount of energy than protein and carbohydrates.

As it is with other macronutrients, the concern should be about the amount and the type of fat that is consumed rather than complete avoidance. You can include foods rich in monosaturated & polyunsaturated fats like avocado and olive oil, which can lower the level of bad cholesterol in the body.

1.22 How to Choose the Right Food

1. 221 FOODS & BEVERAGES TO AVOID

Though most of the food items are desirable concerning a diabetic diet, the ones to avoid are:

- Foods are high in saturated and trans fat.
- Sugary drinks including sugar-laden fruit juices
- Margarine & Shortening
- White Pasta & Rice
- Organ Meats
- Processed Snacks
- Salty & fried foods

1.222 FOODS TO INCLUDE

Before you create any considerable changes in your diet, it is always advisable to consult your doctor and dietician. They can give you a proper understanding of your health condition and how to improve it along with the changes you are adopting. Always go for a healthy eating plan which you can follow through rather than one which is restrictive and hard to follow. Include those foods which you like into your eating plan in such a way that you can have them at least occasionally. When you are deprived of it entirely, it can cause dissatisfaction about your diet and make it hard to follow through. To make a difference, individualize the plans to meet your food preferences, budget, and lifestyle.

Healthy ingredients to be consumed regularly are:

- Whole Fruits
- Non-starchy Vegetables
- Lean meat, poultry & fish
- Healthy Omega-3 fatty acids
- Monosaturated & polyunsaturated fats like those in seeds, nuts, avocado, and olive oil
- Legumes such as beans
- Fatty fishes like Tuna, sardines, and salmon
- Whole Grains such as Oats & Quinoa
- Nuts such as almonds, pecan, and walnuts
- Avocadoes

1.3. FOOD LABELLING & DIABETICS

Proper nutrition is one of the building blocks concerning the effective treatment of diabetics. Therefore, before you buy any manufactured food products, it is significant that you carefully read the ingredient list. Correctly reading food labels can make a difference.

- **Lookout for hearty ingredients & avoid unhealthy ones** - When you are starting, look out first for heart-healthy ingredients that are suitable for the diabetic diet. Then see if you can notice harmful ingredients such as hydrogenated or partially hydrogenated oil in it, which should be avoided by diabetic people at all costs. The ingredient list is usually list based on their weight. The most used ingredients are at the top and the least one at the bottom.

- **Understand the total carbohydrate level** – Rather than looking at the sugar amount listed on the ingredients list, measure the overall carbohydrate level that includes added sugar and fiber also. Focussing only on sugar level can make you miss out on nutritious food like milk and fruits, which are high in sugar. And instead, you might concentrate more on foods that contain artificial sugars.

- **Read sugar-free products carefully** – A sugar-free label means that one serving should contain less than 0.5gm of sugar. So when you compare sugar-free products and normal products, make sure to read carefully. If the sugar-free products have fewer carbohydrates than the standard product, then it should be favoured. On the other hand, if it has more or less the same amount of carbohydrates, then you can decide the product based on taste and price.

Similarly, when you see a no-sugar-added label, it means that it doesn't have any high-sugar ingredients in it, and there was no sugar added during the processing and packaging time. But then, read cautiously as they still can contain carbohydrates.

- **Different serving size** – The serving size given on the packet and the amount we eat might be different. If you are eating twice the amount, then everything gets doubled.
- **Study your daily calorie goals and do the necessary** - The Daily Value listed on food labels is a percentage-based tool based on a 2,000-calorie-a-day diet. The tools benefit you in gauging how much of an exact nutrient one serving of food comprises, paralleled with references for the whole day. 5% or less is low; 20% or more is high. Check and use food products with fats, cholesterol, and sodium percentages on the lower end of the Daily Value while keeping the fiber, vitamins, and minerals percentage on the higher end. If your physician endorses more or less than 2,000 calories a day, you may need to alter the rate as needed — or simply use the percentage as a general frame of reference.

- **Be wary of fat-free products** – Just because the labels say fat-free doesn't mean that it is a healthy product. They still can contain more carbohydrates and calories than the regular product. Compare the food labels and make a choice.

Food labeling can aid in avoiding unhealthy products as well as to understand to good ones. Free foods refer to those food products which have less than 20gm of carbohydrates per serving and as less than 5gm of carbohydrates.

1. 4. GLYCEMIC INDEX AND CONTROLLING DIABETICS

When diagnosed with diabetics, you must classify the food ingredients not only by their caloric content but also based on the glycemic index. Therefore, an understanding of what glycemic index is essential.

Arbohydrates are one of the primary nutrients in food that can raise the sugar level in your body. Glycemic index and glycemic load aid us in understanding what the effect of carbohydrates present in the ingredient has on blood sugar changes. Through this index, we would be able to understand the rate of absorption of carbohydrate-containing foods by the body compared to pure glucose. Apart from the GI index, every ingredient has its energy or calorie content also. The factors that determine it are the number of carbohydrates, fat, and protein it contains.

Glucose with a GI of 100 is the reference point, and relative to it, an indicator gets calculated for other products. The index gets categorized into three groups; high, medium, and low. High GI products are those who have a high content of simple sugars. On the digestion of simple sugars, there will be a significant rise in glucose level and a rapid release of energy. On the other hand, low GI products contain fiber, and therefore, they take a long time to digest because of which the rise in glucose level will be slow and even. Goods with low-glycemic indexes of less than 55% are considered a better choice and are better options for people with diabetics. A moderate GI of 56 to 69% is ok, whereas foods with a glycaemic index of more than 70% are the most harmful.

The glycemic index of foods is variable. The following factors impact its level:

- carbohydrate structure;
- fiber, protein, fat;
- food consistency;
- degree of heat and cooking;
- food absorption rate.

Below is a table showing the Glycemic index of various food products. The values are average and approximate and can change owing to storage conditions, the method of cooking, the original content of carbohydrates in a particular product.

Products with a high GI

Product	GI
White bread	100
Butter buns	95
Pancakes	95
Potato (baked)	95
Rice noodles	95
Canned Apricots	95
Instant rice	90
Honey	90
Instant porridge	85
Carrots (boiled or stewed)	85
Cornflakes	85
Instant rice	90
Mashed potatoes, boiled potatoes	85
Sports drinks (Powerade, Gatorade)	80
Muesli with nuts and raisins	80

Sweet pastries (waffles, donuts)	75
Pumpkin	75
Watermelon	75
Mashed potatoes, boiled potatoes	85
Melon	75
Rice porridge in milk	75
Millet	70
Carrot (raw)	70
Chocolate bar (Mars, Snickers)	70
Milk chocolate	70
Sweet Carbonated Drinks (Pepsi, Coca-Cola)	70
A pineapple	70
Dumplings	70
Soft Wheat Noodles	70
White rice	70
Potato chips	70
Sugar (white or brown)	70
Couscous	70
Manka	70

Products with a medium GI

Product	GI
Wheat flour	65
Orange juice (packaged)	65
Jams and Jams	65
Black yeast bread	65
Marmalade	65
Granola with sugar	65
Raisins	65
Rye bread	65
Jacket boiled potatoes	65
Whole wheat bread	65
Canned vegetables	65
Pasta with cheese	65
Thin pizza with tomatoes and cheese	60
Banana	60
Ice cream	60
Long grain rice	60
Industrial mayonnaise	60

Oatmeal	60
Buckwheat (brown, roasted)	60
Grapes and grape juice	55
Ketchup	55
Spaghetti	55
Canned peaches	55
Shortbread	55

Products with low GI

Product	GI
Cranberries (fresh or frozen)	47
Grapefruit juice (sugar-free)	45
Canned Green Peas	45
Basmati Brown Rice	45
Coconut	45
Grape	45
Orange fresh	45
Whole grain toast	45
Curd	45
Whole-grain cooked breakfasts	43

(without sugar and honey)	
Buckwheat	40
Dried figs	40
Al dente cooked pasta	40
Carrot Juice (Sugar-Free)	40
Dried apricots	40
Prunes	40
Wild (black) rice	35
Chickpeas	35
Fresh apple	35
Bean Meat	35
Dijon mustard	35
Dried tomatoes	35
Fresh green peas	35
Chinese noodles and vermicelli	35
Sesame	35
Fresh orange	35
Fresh plum	35
Fresh quince	35
Soy Sauce (Sugar-Free)	35

Fat-Free Natural Yogurt	35
Fructose ice cream	35
Beans	34
Fresh nectarine	34
Garnet	34
Fresh peach	34
Compote (sugar-free)	34
Tomato juice	33
Yeast	31
Cream 10% fat	30
Soy milk	30
Fresh apricot	30
Brown lentils	30
Fresh grapefruit	30
Green bean	30
Garlic	30
Fresh carrots	30
Fresh beets	30
Jam (sugar-free)	30

Fresh pear	30
Tomato (fresh)	30
Fat-free cottage cheese	30
Yellow lentils	30
Blueberries, lingonberries, blueberries	30
Dark chocolate (over 70% cocoa)	30
Almond milk	30
Milk (any fat content)	30
Passion fruit	30
Pomelo	30
Tangerine fresh	30
A hen	30
Blackberry	20
Cherry	25
Green lentils	25
Golden Beans	25
Fresh raspberries	25
Red Ribes	25
Strawberry wild-strawberry	25

Pumpkin seeds	25
Gooseberry	25
Soya flour	25
Kefir non-fat	25
Cherries	22
Peanut Butter (Sugar-Free)	20
Artichoke	20
Eggplant	20
Soy yogurt	20
Almond	20
Broccoli	20
Cabbage	20
Cashew	15
Celery	15
Bran	15
Brussels sprouts	15
Cauliflower	15
Chilli	15
Fresh cucumber	15

Hazelnuts, pine nuts, pistachios, walnuts	15
Asparagus	15
Ginger	15
Mushrooms	15
Squash	15
Onion	15
Pesto	15
Leek	15
Olives	15
Peanut	15
Pickled and Pickled Cucumbers	15
Rhubarb	15
Tofu (bean curd)	15
Soybean	15
Spinach	15
Avocado	10
Leaf salad	9
Parsley, basil, vanillin, cinnamon, oregano	5

Many factors can change the glycemic index of the product, which must be taken into account when creating a diet with a low GI.

Some examples to illustrate it are the following:

• Storage period and maturity of starchy products. For example, an unripe banana has a low GI of 40, but after it ripens and softens, the GI increases to 65. When ripening, apples also increase GI, but not so fast;

• Heating cooked food after storage in the refrigerator lowers GI

• Cooking escalates GI. For example, boiled carrots have a GI of 50, while in raw form, it does not exceed 20 as the starch contained in carrots gels when heated.

• Most of the industrial products get heat treatment for gelatinizing starchy products. For this reason, corn flakes, instant mashed potatoes, cereals for cooked breakfasts have a very high GI - 85 and 95, respectively.

• Numerous products include "corn starch."The GI of cornstarch is close to 100 and can increase glycemia. So avoid it at all costs.

• Pasta should always be slightly undercooked so that they crack somewhat on the teeth. If you cook pasta for 15-20 minutes, the gelatinization of starch will increase, and GI will increase to 70. If you cook spaghetti (even from white flour)

using al dente (slightly undercooked) and serve cold, for example, in a salad, then GI will be only 35.
- Extended storage of certain products containing starch adds to the reduction of GI. Warm, freshly baked bread will have a much higher GI than the one that has cooled, and the more than the one that has dried.
- Use as many vegetables as possible in your diet. Their low GI makes it possible not only to increase the reserves of vitamins and minerals but also to eat in any quantity. Besides, vegetables lower the GI of other foods if eaten together. The fiber in vegetables significantly reduces blood sugar, as it takes a lot of energy to digest it.
- Choose cooking methods that help lower your GI. The stronger the starch-containing product gets boiled (porridge, pasta, potatoes, cereals), the higher the GI.
- Grinding food products like vegetables raise their GI. For example, a piece of meat has a lower GI than meatballs. Any crushing hastens the digestion, which means less energy is needed. Therefore, do not try to grind vegetables for salads too finely. Raw carrots are healthier than grated and even more so than boiled.
- It is not that important to peel natural vegetables and fruits since it can lengthen the digestion process and lower GI.
- Spoon a bit of vegetable oil to salads and other dishes, as all oils reduce down the digestion process, damage the absorption of sugars, and lower GI.

- Separation of food products based on micronutrients is not necessary as proteins can dawdle down the intake of carbohydrates, lower glucose, and lower GI. In turn, carbohydrates are essential for the absorption of proteins. Therefore, in a diet, it is necessary to mix a protein dish with a vegetable dish.
- In the daily diet, it is vital to lower the GI with each meal. In the morning, it can be quite high, at lunch - dishes with medium GI, and for dinner - only low GI. During a night's rest, energy consumption is at a lower level, which means that everything eaten at night gets converted to body fat.

However, diet planning and metabolic normalization in a patient with diabetes should not be decided based on glycemic index tables only. The system does not fully appraise carbohydrate-free foods. Therefore, when it comes to diet, you need to look at the shelf life of food products, the method of cooking, which can significantly affect GI. You also need to consider that the menu should take into account age, lifestyle, and the general state of human health.

It is not that the products with a high GI are detrimental, but instead, it is their unwarranted and uninhibited consumption that causes problems. For example, if you have worked hard doing physical activity for more than an hour, then a high GI will go to restore energy. Instead, if you eat these products in front of the TV, then body fat will rise by leaps and bounds.

Regular consumption, though, can cause problems as they can disrupt the body's metabolic process. Because of the surge in glucose after their use, it can cause a chronic feeling of hunger while creating the formation of fat in high-risk areas like the abdomen.

Now regarding the difference between glycemic index and glycemic load is that the index is a standardized measurement. In contrast, the glycemic load gives us a picture of the real-life portion size. Therefore, the glycemic load is a better tool.

CHAPTER 2

2.1. MEAL PLANNING & DIABETIC MANAGEMENT

Meal planning can go a long way in maintaining the proper level of blood sugar for diabetic patients. You should have the confidence you will stick on to those healthy changes in your lifestyle and diet. Once you have got a grasp, the whole process will become easier. A positive attitude can make all the change.

The 4-week meal plan is a straightforward map that can help you right from the start of a month or whenever you are starting. The meal plan is full of delicious and nourishing recipes that are good in all aspects while being simple and easy to make. Plan and concoct as much as you can as they set the foundation.

2.21 Week Meal Plan for Non-Vegetarians

WEEK 1

Day 1
1 serving of Egg Cups + 1 oz. Pistachios + Green Tea – Breakfast (298kcal, 66.85gm fat, 11.72g protein & 8.17gm carbs)
1 serving of Cherry Pork Tenderloin + 1 serving of Grilled Broccoli - Lunch (466Kcal, 25.3gm fat, 41gm proteins & 18gm carbs)
1 serving of Salmon with Asparagus + 1 serving of roasted Green Beans – Dinner (442Kcal, 31.3gm fat, 33.5gm proteins & 5.4gm carbs)
Chocolate Keto Bombs – Dessert.
Day 2
1 serving of Cream Cheese Pancakes + 1 cup of Raspberries – Breakfast (407Kcal, 29.8gm fat, 18.5gm proteins & 9gm carbs)
1 serving of Tuna Tartare + 2 Cucumbers, sliced – Lunch

(280kcal + 15.6gmfat, 27.8proteins & 2.6gm carbs)

1 serving of Chicken Casserole – Dinner (612Kcal, 56gm fat, 36gm proteins & 6gm carbs)

Bounty Bars – Dessert (200Kcal, 14.6gm fat, 1gm proteins & 6gm carbs).

Day 3

3 serving of Cloud Bread + 3 tbsp. Butter – Breakfast (408Kcal, 39gm fat, 2.36gm Proteins & 1.3gm carbs)

1 serving of Grilled Salmon + 1 serving of Steamed Asparagus – Lunch (302Kcal, 9gm Fat, 46gm proteins & 8.2gm carb)

1 serving of Cobb Salad + 1 serving of Mashed Cauliflower – Dinner (407Kcal, 28.5gm Fat, 29.8gm proteins & 9gm carbs)

Raspberry Ice Cream – Dessert.

Day 4

1 serving of Bagels + 3 tbsp. Peanut Butter – Breakfast (612Kcal, 52gm fat, 31.5gm Proteins & 15gm carbs)

1 serving of Broccoli Bacon Salad + 1 serving of Barbeque Diabetic Chicken – Lunch (556.7Kcal, 32.32gm fat, 48.24gm proteins & 11.3gm carbs)

1 serving of Creamed Spinach + 1 serving of Roasted

Meat – Dinner (439Kcal, 30.6gm Fat, 35gm proteins & 4gm carbs)

Cookie Dough – Dessert (148Kcal, 14gm fat, 6gm proteins & 4gm carbs).

Day 5

1 serving of Granola + 1 cup of Yoghurt + 100gm Berries – Breakfast (484Kcal, 34.3gm Fat, 16.2gm proteins & 14.6gm of carbs)

1 serving of Chicken Soup + 1 serving of Zoodles – Lunch (360Kcal, 22gm fat, 29gm Proteins & 13gm carbs)

1 serving of Shrimp in Garlic Butter + 1 serving of Shirataki Noodles – Dinner(327Kcal, 20gm fat, 27gm protein & 9gm carbs)

Chia Pudding – Dessert (15Kcal, 10gm fat, 5gm proteins &1.5gm carbs).

Day 6

1 serving of Pancakes + 1 serving of Low-Carb Sweetener Syrup – Breakfast (278Kcal, 23gm fat, 9gm proteins & 1.5gm carbs)

1 serving of Beef Stew + 1 serving of Green Salad – Lunch (388Kcal, 25gm fat, 24.1gm Proteins & 15gm carbs)

1 serving of Seared Tuna Steak + 1 serving of Parmesan

Roasted Broccoli – Dinner (337kcal, 13.6gm fat, 45.5gm proteins & 13.6gm carbs)
Chocolate Ice Cream – Dessert (127Kcal, 2.6gm fat, 20gm proteins & 5.6gm carbs).
Day 7
1 serving of Waffles + 1 serving of Berries – Breakfast (353Kcal, 23.5gm fat, 10.1gm Proteins & 20gm carbs)
1 serving of Meatloaf + ½ Baked Sweet Potato – Lunch (562Kcal, 25gm fat, 17.24gm Proteins & 24.35gm carbs)
1 serving of Cheesy Cauliflower Gratin + 1 serving of Grilled Chicken – Dinner (586Kcal, 73gm fat, 50gm proteins & 9gm carbs)
Strawberry Popsicles – Dessert.

WEEK 2

Day 1
1 serving of Quinoa Porridge + 50 gm. of Almonds – Breakfast (448Kcal, 30gm fat, 28.7gm proteins & 33gm carbs)
1 serving of Pulled Pork + 1 cup Lettuce Leaves – Lunch (500Kcal, 15.1gm fat, 48gm Proteins & 5gm carbs)

1 serving of Strawberry Spinach Salad + 1 serving of Quinoa – Dinner (477Kcal, 20gm Fat, 22.14gm of proteins & 43gm carbs)

Chocolate Peanut Butter Blondie's – Dessert (265Kcal, 23.6gm fat, 8.72gm proteins & 8.5gm carbs).

Day 2

1 serving of Broiled Grapefruit + 1 cup of Yoghurt – Breakfast (257Kcal, 8gm fat, 9.5gm Proteins & 37.4gm of carbs)

1 serving of Black Bean Soup + 1 serving of Spinach Salad– Lunch (430kcal, 19gm fat, 25.8gm proteins & 25gm carbs)

1 serving of Lamb Chops + 1 serving of Cauliflower Rice – Dinner (383Kcal, 18.2gm Fat, 48.3gm proteins & 4.2 gm. carbs)

Vanilla Bean Ice Cream – Dessert (172Kcal, 15.2gm fat, 4.1gm proteins & 5.2gm carbs).

Day 3

1 serving of Egg Scramble with Beans – Breakfast (480.5Kcal, 15gm fat, 32gm proteins & 34gm carbs)

1 serving of Grilled Vegetables with Kabobs + 1 serving of couscous salad – Lunch (443Kcal, 20gm fat, 31gm proteins & 31gm carbs)

1 serving of Adobo Chicken + 1 serving of shredded Carrot Salad – Dinner (325Kcal, 11.5gm fat, 3.9gm proteins & 25gm carbs)

Chocolate Mousse – Dessert (218Kcal, 23gm fat, 2gm proteins & 3gm carbs).

Day 4

1 serving of Oatmeal with Sweet Potatoes + 1 serving of Walnuts – Breakfast (364Kcal, 26gm of fats, 11.4gm of proteins & 21gm carbs)

1 serving of Herbed Chicken Sausage Patties + 1 serving of Hearty Green Salad – Lunch (501kcal, 15.4gm fat, 34.4gm proteins & 35.5gm carbs)

1 serving of Shrimp & Avocado Salad + 1 serving of Toastada – Dinner (345Kcal, 16gm Fat, 32gm proteins & 15gm carbs)

Chocolate Coconut Balls – Dessert (134Kcal, 7gm fat, 2gm proteins & 21gm carbs).

Day 5

1 serving of Banana Egg Oatmeal + 1 serving of Berries – Breakfast (257Kcal, 10.1gm Fat, 8.3gm proteins & 30.7gm carbs)

1 serving of Garden Pasta Salad + 1 serving of Baked Asparagus – Lunch (294Kcal, 9.3gm fat, 20.1gm proteins

& 29gm carbs)

1 serving of Adobo Chicken + 1 serving of Citrus Green Salad – Dinner (397Kcal, 49gm Fat, 35gm proteins & 7.5gm carbs)

Low-Carb Cheesecake – Dessert (600Kcal, 54gm fat, 14gm proteins & 7gm carbs).

Day 6

1 serving of Nut & Seed Cereal + 1 Pear – Breakfast (378Kcal, 15gm fat, 13gm proteins & 41gm carbs)

1 serving of Potato Soup + 1 serving of Cabbage & Carrot Salad – Lunch (660kcal, 10gm Fat, 8.5gm proteins & 26gm carbs)

1 serving of Butter Chicken + 1 serving of Cauliflower Rice – Dinner (410Kcal, 27gm Fat, 28.5gm proteins & 9gm carbs)

Keto Brownies – Dessert (116Kcal, 11gm fat, 2gm proteins & 3gm carbs).

Day 7

1 serving of Arugula Smoothie + 1 cup Berries + Cheese – Breakfast (434Kcal, 25gm Fat, 19.6gm proteins & 28gm carbs)

1 serving of Lentil Stew + 1 serving of Salsa Verde – Lunch (333Kcal, 7.5gm fat, 19.1gm Proteins & 32gm carbs)

1 serving of Cream of Asparagus Soup + 1 serving of Green Salad – Dinner (101Kcal, 3.2gm fat, 15gm proteins & 10.2gm carbs)

Keto Vanilla Mug Cake – Dessert (342Kcal, 27gm fat, 9gm proteins & 4.5gm carbs)

WEEK 3

Day 1

1 serving of Blueberry Muffins + 1 tbsp. Nut Butter – Breakfast (405Kcal, 35gm fat, 14gm proteins & 7gm carbs)

1 serving of Cheeseburger Squash Casserole – Lunch (431Kcal, 28.8gm fat, 30.5 Proteins & 5gm carbs)

1 serving of Vegetable Soup + 1 serving of Grilled Chicken – Dinner (363Kcal, 8.5gm Fat, 59gm proteins & 8gm carbs)

Key Lime Pie – Dessert (325Kcal, 32gm fat, 4gm proteins & 5gm carbs).

Day 2

1 serving of Almond Flour Porridge + 1 cup Berries – Breakfast (281Kcal, 18gm fat, 9.5gm proteins & 3.5gm carbs)

1 serving of Zucchini Noodles with Pesto + ½ of 1 Avocado sliced – Lunch (546Kcal, 49gm fat, 9gm proteins & 9gm carbs)

1 serving of Baked Chicken Legs + 1 serving of Spicy Dipping Sauce – Dinner (302Kcal, 24gm fat, 6gm proteins & 18gm carbs)

Lemon Cookies – Dessert (150Kcal, 27gm fat, 9gm proteins & 4.5gm carbs).

Day 3

1 serving of Banana Bread + 1 serving of Walnuts – Breakfast (333Kcal, 28.3gm fat, 9.3gm proteins & 4.8gm carbs)

1 serving of Seafood Chowder – Lunch (795Kcal, 69gm fat, 37gm proteins & 6gm Carbs)

1 serving of Chicken Piccata + 1 serving of Roasted Edamame – Dinner (442Kcal, 21gm Fat, 46gm proteins & 6gm carbs)

Chocolate Zucchini Cake – Dessert (265Kcal, 23.6gm fat, 8.5gm proteins & 8gm Carbs).

Day 4

1 serving of Pumpkin Pancakes + 1 serving of Almond Butter – Breakfast (321Kcal, 24.4gm fat, 14.2gm proteins & 5.6gm carbs)

1 serving of Cauliflower Fried Rice + 1 serving of Roasted Salmon – Lunch (305Kcal, 15.3gm fat, 31gm proteins & 7.7gm carbs)

1 serving of Stuffed Peppers + 1 serving of Crunchy Salad – Dinner (234Kcal, 15gm Fat, 17gm proteins & 6gm carbs)

Chocolate Peanut Butter Cookies – Dessert (265Kcal, 23.6gm fat, 8.72gm proteins & 8.5gm carbs).

Day 5

1 serving of Baked Avocado Egg + 1 serving of Shredded Cheese – Breakfast (385Kcal, 30gm fat, 20gm proteins & 2.3 gm carbs)

1 serving of Broccoli Cheddar Soup + 1 serving of Vinegar Fresh Coleslaw – Lunch (318Kcal, 27gm fat, 8gm proteins & 8gm carbs)

1 serving of Cobb Salad + 1 serving of Mashed Cauliflower – Dinner (400Kcal, 28.5gm Fat, 5.2gm proteins & 6.4gm carbs)

Chocolate Mousse – Dessert (218Kcal, 23gm fat, 5.2gm proteins & 6.4gm carbs).

Day 6

1 serving of Cauliflower Hash Browns + 1 serving of Scrambled Eggs – Breakfast (430Kcal, 37gm fat, 13gm proteins & 8.6gm carbs)

1 serving of Roasted Green Beans + 1 serving of Shirataki Noodles – Lunch (93Kcal, 5gm fat, 7gm proteins & 8gm carbs)

1 serving of Beef Chili + 1 serving of Sliced Avocadoes – Dinner (309Kcal, 17gm fat, 34gm proteins & 5gm carbs)

Key Lime Pie – Dessert (325Kcal, 32gm fat, 4gm proteins & 5gm carbs).

Day 7

1 serving of Avocado Toast + 3 slices of Bacon Slices – Breakfast (621Kcal, 50gm fat, 29.5gm proteins & 2.7gm carbs)

1 serving of Kale Salad + 1 serving of Cooked Tofu – Lunch (336Kcal, 26gm fat, 16gm Proteins & 8gm carbs)

1 serving of Stuffed Mushrooms + 1 serving of Roasted Broccoli – Dinner (144Kcal, 9.5gm fat, 8gm proteins & 6.3gm carbs)

Chia Seed Pudding – Dessert (151Kcal, 10gm fat, 5gm proteins & 1.5gm carbs).

WEEK 4

Day 1

1 serving of Vegetable Frittata + 1 serving of Salad Greens – Breakfast (212Kcal, 15.4gm fat, 12.9gm proteins & 3.7gm carbs)

1 serving of Pimento Cheese Balls – Lunch (651Kcal, 52gm fat, 41gm proteins & 1 gm Carbs)

1 serving of Chicken Enchilada Soup – Dinner (585Kcal, 52.3gm fat, 16gm proteins & 9gm carbs)

Oats Coffee Smoothie – Dessert (251Kcal, 15.1gm fat, 20.3gm proteins & 6.9gm carbs).

Day 2

1 serving of Butter Coffee – Breakfast (334Kcal, 38gm fat, 1gm proteins & 0gm carbs)

1 serving of Cauliflower Pizza + ¼ cup Extra Cheese + 1 serving of Olives – Lunch (248Kcal, 19.1gm fat, 14.3gm proteins & 6gm carbs)

1 serving of Strawberry Spinach Salad + 1 serving of Quinoa – Dinner (477Kcal, 20gm Fat, 22.14gm proteins & 43gm carbs)

Strawberry Cheesecake Smoothie – Dessert (347Kcal, 24gm fat, 17.5gm proteins & 10.05gm carbs).

Day 3

1 serving of Green Detox Juice + 2 tbsp. of MCT Oil – Breakfast (417Kcal, 46gm fat, 12.3gm proteins & 3.6gm carbs)

1 serving of Cauliflower Mac & Cheese + 1 Ham Slice – Lunch (417Kcal, 28gmfat, 29gm proteins & 8gm carbs)

1 serving of Pumpkin Soup – Dinner (610Kcal, 57.9gm fat, 14.4gm proteins & 7.7gm Carbs)

Cinnamon Roll Smoothie – Dessert (145Kcal, 3.25gm fat, 26.5gm proteins & 1.6gm Carbs).

Day 4

1 serving of Bacon & Egg + 1 serving of Plum Tomatoes, chopped – Breakfast (288Kcal, 22.2gm fat, 15.8gm proteins & 3.4gm carbs)

1 serving of Chicken Soup + 1 serving of Zoodles – Lunch (370Kcal, 22gm fat, 29gm Proteins & 13gm carbs)

1 serving of Easy Egg Salad & 1 serving of Lettuce Leaves – Dinner (181Kcal, 14.15gm Fat, 11.36gm proteins & 2.42gm carbs)

Chocolate Keto Bombs – Dessert (84Kcal, 8.2gm fat, 2gm proteins & 1.6gm carbs).

Day 5

1 serving of Pumpkin Bread + 1 tbsp. of Cream Cheese – Breakfast (265.8Kcal, 23gm Fat, 8.9gm proteins & 4.8gm carbs)

1 serving of Strawberry Spinach Salad + 1 oz. of Walnuts – Lunch (440Kcal, 34.5gm Fat, 18.3gm proteins & 10gm carbs)

1 serving of Baked Cod with Lemon – Dinner (440Kcal, 22.1gm fat, 46.8gm proteins & 14.5gm carbs)

Raspberry Ice Cream – Dessert (183Kcal, 16gm fat, 1gm proteins & 3gm carbs).

Day 6

1 serving of Berry Mint Smoothie + 1 tbsp. Flax Seeds + – Breakfast (388Kcal, 9.9gm Fat, 7.9gm proteins & 16gm carbs)

1 serving of Thai Tofu Curry + 1 serving of Cauliflower Rice – Lunch (345Kcal, 28gm Fat, 14gm proteins & 12gm carbs)

1 serving of Chicken Casserole – Dinner (612Kcal, 56gm fat, 36gm proteins & 6gm carbs)

Strawberry Popsicles – Dessert (73Kcal, 1gm fat, 3.5gm proteins & 12gm carbs).

Day 7
1 serving of Blackberry Smoothie + 1 serving of Almonds – Breakfast (439Kcal, 31gm Fat, 17gm proteins & 12gm carbs)
1 serving of Five-Spice Chicken Drumsticks + 1 serving of Cabbage Stir Fry – Lunch (162Kcal, 7.7gm fat, 5.6gm proteins & 14gm carbs)
1 serving of Greek Broccoli Salad + 1 serving of Grilled Beef – Dinner (522Kcal, 36gm Fat, 34gm proteins & 12gm carbs)
Chocolate Fudge – Dessert (155Kcal, 15.5gm fat, 1.87gm proteins & 11gm carbs).

2.22 Week Meal Plan for Vegetarians

WEEK 1

Day 1
1 serving of Cream Cheese Pancakes + 1 cup of Raspberries – Breakfast (407Kcal, 29.8gm fat, 18.5gm proteins & 9gm carbs) 1 serving of Zucchini Noodles with Pesto + ½ of 1 Avocado, sliced – Lunch (546Kcal, 49gm fat, 9gm proteins & 9gm carbs)
1 serving of Cauliflower Pizza + 1 serving of Olives – Dinner (138Kcal, 10.1gm fat, 8.3gm proteins& 6.1gm carbs)
Chocolate Keto Fat Bombs – Desserts (84Kcal, 8.2gm fat, 2gm proteins & 1.6gm carbs).
Day 2
1 serving of Strawberry Smoothie + 1 oz. Chia Seeds – Breakfast (305Kcal, 15gm fat, 20.7gm proteins & 13gm carbs)
1 serving of Cauliflower Fried Rice + 1 serving of Tofu – Lunch (198Kcal, 12.6gm fat, 12gm proteins & 8gm carbs)
1 serving of Roasted Green Beans + 1 serving of Mashed Cauliflower – Dinner (166Kcal, 13.5gm fat, 8.5gm proteins & 4.5gm carbs)

Chia Pudding – Dessert (151Kcal, 10gm fat, 5gm proteins & 1.5gm carbs).

Day 3

3 serving of Cloud Bread + 3 tbsp. Butter – Breakfast (408Kcal, 39gm fat, 2.36gm proteins & 1.3gm carbs)

1 serving of Pumpkin Soup – Lunch (610Kcal, 57.9gm fat, 14.4gm proteins & 7.7gm carbs)

1 serving of Greek Broccoli Salad + 1 serving of Grilled Vegetables – Dinner (357Kcal, 25gm fats, 12gm proteins & 17.9gmcarbs)

Chocolate Avocado Pudding – Dessert (199Kcal, 17.8gm fat, 2.9gm proteins & 3.6gm Carbs).

Day 4

1 serving of Coconut Spinach Smoothie – Breakfast (251Kcal, 15.1gm fat, 20.3gm Proteins & 10.9gm carbs)

1 serving of Stuffed Mushrooms + 1 serving of Roasted Broccoli – Lunch (144Kcal, 9.5gm fat, 8gm proteins & 6.3gm carbs)

1 serving of Potato Soup + 1 serving of Cabbage Salad – Dinner (660Kcal, 27gm fat, 28.5gm proteins & 9gm carbs)

Raspberry Ice Cream – Dessert (183Kcal, 16gm fat, 1gm

proteins & 3gm carbs).

Day 5

1 serving of Bagels + 1 serving of Nut Butter – Breakfast (612Kcal, 51gm fat, 31.5gm Proteins & 15gm carbs)

1 serving of Kale Salad + 1 serving of Asian Tofu – Lunch (336Kcal, 26gm fat, 16 gm Proteins & 8gm carbs)

1 serving of Cheesy Cauliflower Gratin – Dinner (421Kcal, 37gm carbs, 19gm proteins & 3gm carbs)

Cookie Dough – Dessert (74Kcal, 6.9gm fat, 1.9gm proteins & 3gm carbs).

Day 6

1 serving of Veggie Smoothie + 1 oz. Pistachios – Breakfast (328Kcal, 22.65gm fat, 8gm proteins & 3gm carbs)

1 serving of Greek Salad + Low-carb Vegetable Soup – Lunch (196Kcal, 11gm fat, 6gm Proteins & 14gm carbs)

1 serving of Strawberry Spinach Salad + 1 serving of Quinoa – Dinner (477Kcal, 20gm Fat, 22.14gm proteins & 43gm carbs)

Keto Brownies – Dessert (116Kcal, 11gm fat, 2gm proteins & 3gm carbs).

Day 7
1 serving of Granola Bars + 1 serving of Yoghurt + 100gm Berries – Breakfast (484Kcal, 34.3gm fat, 16.2gm proteins & 14.6gm carbs)
1 serving of Broccoli Cheddar Soup + 1 serving of Vinegar Coleslaw– Lunch (318Kcal, 27gm fat, 8gm proteins & 8gm carbs)
1 serving of Easy Egg Salad + 1 serving of Lettuce Leaves – Dinner (181Kcal, 14.15gm Fat, 11.36 gm of proteins & 2.42gm carbs)
Keto Lime Pie – Dessert (325Kcal, 32gm fat, 4gm proteins & 5gm carbs).

WEEK 2

Day 1
1 serving of Green Smoothie + 1 oz. Chia Seeds – Breakfast (262Kcal, 11gm fat, 6gm Proteins & 28gm carbs)
1 serving of Garden Pasta Salad + 1 serving of Baked Asparagus – Lunch (294Kcal, 9.3gm fat, 20.1gm proteins & 29gm carbs)
1 serving of Garlic Mashed Cauliflower + 1 serving of Greek Salad – Dinner (243Kcal, 18gm fat, 10gm proteins

& 15gm carbs)

Vanilla Bean Ice Cream – Dessert (172Kcal, 15.2gm fat, 4.1gm proteins & 5.2gm carbs).

Day 2

1 serving of Banana Egg Oatmeal + 1 serving of Berries – Breakfast (257Kcal, 10.1gm Fat, 8.3gm proteins & 30gm carbs)

1 serving of Black Bean Soup + 1 serving of Spinach Salad – Lunch (430Kcal, 19gm Fat, 25.8gm proteins & 25gm carbs)

1 serving of Creamed Spinach + 1 serving of Oven Roasted Veggies – Dinner (425Kcal, 33gm fat, 6gm proteins & 23gm carbs)

Strawberry Popsicles – Dessert (73Kcal, 0.5gm fat, 3.5gm proteins & 12gm carbs).

Day 3

1 serving of Peanut Butter Banana Smoothie + 1 serving of Sugar-Free Chocolate Chips – Breakfast (272Kcal, 13.5gm fat, 11gm proteins & 23gm carbs)

1 serving of Thai Tofu Curry + 1 serving of Cauliflower Rice – Lunch (343Kcal, 27.3gm Fat, 14gm proteins & 10gm carbs)

1 serving of Stuffed Mushrooms + 1 serving of Oven Roasted Brussels Sprouts – Dinner (144Kcal, 9.5gm fat, 8gm proteins & 6.3gm carbs)

Chocolate Zucchini Cake – Dessert (265Kcal, 23.6gm fat, 8.72gm proteins & 8.5gm Carbs).

Day 4

1 serving of Quinoa Porridge + 1 oz. Toasted Almonds – Breakfast (448Kcal, 30gm fat, 28.7gm proteins & 33gm carbs)

1 serving of Cream of Asparagus Soup + 1 serving of Simple Green Salad – Lunch (109Kcal, 7gm fat, 6gm proteins & 6gm carbs)

1 serving of Kale Salad + 1 serving of Sesame Garlic Tofu – Dinner (336Kcal, 26gm fat, 16gm proteins & 8gm carbs)

Low- Carb Cheesecake – Dessert (600Kcal, 54gm fat,14gm proteins & 7gm carbs).

Day 5

1 serving of Nut & Seed Cereal + 1 Pear – Breakfast (378Kcal, 15gm fat, 13gm proteins & 40gm carbs)

1 serving of Tomato Gazpacho + 1 serving of Cauliflower Salad – Lunch (475Kcal, 38.1gm fat, 15gm proteins & 18gm carbs)

1 serving of Pumpkin Soup – Dinner (610Kcal, 58gm fat, 14.4gm proteins & 7gm Carbs)

Chocolate Fudge – Dessert (154Kcal, 15.5gm fat, 1.8gm proteins & 10.7gm carbs).

Day 6

1 serving of Broiled Grapefruit +1 serving of Yoghurt – Breakfast (257Kcal, 8gm fat, 9.5gm proteins & 37.4gm carbs)

1 serving of Cauliflower Soup + 1 serving of Cheese, shredded – Lunch (306Kcal, 25gm fat, 10gm proteins & 8gm carbs)

1 serving of Zucchini Noodles with Pesto + 1 serving of Tomato Soup – Dinner (488Kcal, 22.7gm fat, 10.gm proteins & 8.3gm carbs)

Chocolate Ice Cream – Dessert (127Kcal, 2.2gm fat, 20.1 gm proteins & 5.6gm carbs).

Day 7

1 serving of Matcha Green Smoothie + 1 serving of Almonds – Breakfast (393Kcal, 57gm fat, 20.1gm proteins & 4.5gm carbs)

1 serving of Cabbage Slaw + 1 serving of Shirataki Noodles – Lunch (130Kcal, 7gm fat, 1.8gm proteins & 14gm carbs)

1 serving of Broccoli Cheddar Soup + 1 serving of Vinegar Coleslaw – Dinner (318Kcal, 27gm fat, 8gm proteins & 8gm carbs)

Chocolate Coconut Balls – Dessert (134Kcal, 7gm fat, 2gm proteins & 21gm carbs).

WEEK 3

Day 1

1 serving of Avocado Smoothie + 1 serving of Cashews – Breakfast (371Kcal, 29gm fat 7.2gm proteins & 22gm carbs)

1 serving of Lentil Stew + 1 serving of Salsa Verde – Lunch (333Kcal, 7.5gm fat, 19.1gm Proteins & 32gm carbs)

1 serving of Green Detox Juice + 2 tbsp. MCT Oil – Dinner (297Kcal, 17.6gm fat, 12.3gm proteins & 18gm carbs)

Keto Vanilla Mug Cake – Dessert (342Kcal, 27gm fat, 9gm proteins & 4.5gm carbs).

Day 2

1 serving of Pumpkin Pancakes + 1 serving of Almond Butter – Breakfast (321Kcal, 24.4gm fat, 14.2gm proteins & 5.6gm carbs)

1 serving of Cauliflower Pizza + ¼ cup Extra Cheese + 1 serving of Olives – Lunch (248Kcal, 19.1gm of fat, 14.3gm proteins & 6gm carbs)
1 serving of Avocado Turmeric Smoothie + 3 tbsp. Mixed Nuts – Dinner (502.kcal, 46.4gm fat, 9.7gm proteins & 7.2gm carbs)
Keto Chocolate Fat Bombs – Dessert (84Kcal, 8.2gm fat, 2gm proteins & 1.6gm carbs).
Day 3
1 serving of Orange Carrot Smoothie + 2 tbsp. Collagen Powder – Breakfast (262Kcal, 7gm fats, 39gm proteins & 10gm carbs)
1 serving of Strawberry Spinach Salad + 1 serving of Quinoa – Lunch (477Kcal, 20gm Fat, 22.14gm proteins & 43gm carbs)
1 serving of Veggie Smoothie + 1 serving of Mixed Nuts – Dinner (439kcal, 33.8gm Fat, 11.2gm proteins & 20.1gmcarbs)
Bounty Bars – Dessert (100Kcal, 7.3gm fat, 0.5gm proteins & 6gm carbs).
Day 4
1 serving of Almond Flour Porridge + 1 cup Berries – Breakfast (281Kcal, 18gm fat, 9.5gm proteins & 3.5gm

carbs)

1 serving of Black Bean Soup + 1 Green Leafy Salad – Lunch (320Kcal, 9.4gm fat, 3.8gm proteins & 26gm carbs)

1 serving of Zucchini Noodles with Pesto +1/2 of 1 Avocado, sliced – Dinner (546kcal, 49gm fat, 9 gm proteins & 9gm carbs)

Raspberry Lemonade – Dessert (107Kcal, 1gm fat, 1.7gm proteins & 20gm carbs).

Day 5

1 serving of Tropical Smoothie + 2 tbsp. Chia Seeds +1 oz. Walnuts – Breakfast (360Kcal, 28gm fat, 9.3gm proteins & 9gm carbs)

1 serving of Roasted Green Beans + 1 serving of Shirataki Noodles – Lunch (93Kcal, 5gm fat, 7gm proteins & 8gm carbs)

1 serving of Cauliflower Fried Rice + 1 serving of Ginger Tofu – Dinner (198Kcal, 12.6gm fat, 12gm proteins & 8gm carbs)

Peanut Butter Cookies – Dessert (140Kcal, 10.4gm fats, 5.8gm proteins & 2.8gm Carbs).

Day 6

1 serving of Avocado Toast + 1 Tomato, chopped –

Breakfast (476Kcal, 37.8gm fat, 18.3gm proteins & 4.5gm carbs)

1 serving of Greek Broccoli Salad + 1serving of Grilled Vegetables – Lunch (357Kcal, 25.6gm fat, 12gm proteins & 17gm carbs)

1 serving of Vegetable Soup + 1 serving of Greek Salad – Dinner (399Kcal, 24gm fat, 21gm proteins & 14gm carbs)

Keto Brownies – Dessert (116Kcal,11gm fat, 2gm proteins & 3gm carbs).

Day 7

1 serving of Key Lime Smoothie + 1 serving of Almonds – Breakfast (344Kcal, 15.2gm Fat, 9.6gm proteins & 10gm carbs)

1 serving of Cheesy Cauliflower Gratin – Lunch (421kcal, 37gm fat, 19gm proteins & 3gm carbs)

1 serving of Greek Salad – Dinner (246Kcal, 14.5gm fat, 9.4gm proteins & 16gm carbs)

Cookie Dough – Dessert (74Kcal, 6.9gm fat, 1.9gm proteins & 3gm carbs).

WEEK 4

Day 1

1 serving of Vegetable Frittata + 1 serving of Salad Greens – Breakfast (212Kcal, 15.4gm fat, 12.9gm proteins & 3.7gm carbs)

1 serving of Pumpkin Soup – Lunch (610Kcal, 57.9gm fat, 14.4gm proteins & 7.7gm Carbs)

1 serving of Cream of Asparagus + 1 serving of Tangy Green Salad – Dinner (101Kcal, 3.2gm fat, 15gm proteins & 10.2gm carbs)

Strawberry Cheesecake Smoothie – Dessert (347Kcal, 24gm fat, 17.5gm proteins & 10.5gm carbs).

Day 2

1 serving of Butter Coffee – Breakfast (334Kcal, 38gm fat & 1gm proteins) 1 serving of Broccoli Cheddar Soup

1 serving of Vegetable Vinegar Coleslaw – Lunch (318Kcal, 27gm fat, 8gm proteins & 8gm carbs)

1 serving of Strawberry Spinach Salad + 1 cup of Quinoa – Dinner (488Kcal, 20gm fat, 22gm proteins & 43gm carbs)

Avocado Turmeric Smoothie – Dessert (232Kcal, 22.1gm fat, 1.7gm proteins & 4.1gm Carbs).

Day 3	
1 serving of Pumpkin Pancakes + 1 serving of Almond Butter – Breakfast (321Kcal, 24.4gm fat, 14.2gm proteins & 5.6gm carbs)	
1 serving of Cauliflower Mac & Cheese – Lunch (292Kcal, 23gm fat, 11gm proteins & 7gm carbs)	
1 serving of Vegetable Soup + 1 serving of Greek Salad – Dinner (399Kcal, 24gm fat, 21gm proteins & 14gm carbs)	
Cinnamon Roll Smoothie – Dessert (145Kcal, 3.25gm fat, 26.5gm proteins & 1.6gm Carbs).	
Day 4	
1 serving of Blueberry Muffins + 1 serving of Nut Butter – Breakfast (405Kcal, 35gm fat, 14gm proteins & 7gm carbs)	
1 serving of Tomato Gazpacho + 1 serving of Grilled Cheese Rolls – Lunch (249Kcal, 11.1gm fat, 4.7gm proteins & 7gm carbs)	
1 serving of Easy Egg Salad + 1 cup of Shredded Lettuce Leaves – Dinner (170Kcal, 20.1gm fat, 10.05gm proteins & 2gm carbs)	
Blackberry Smoothie – Dessert (275Kcal, 17gm fat, 11gm proteins & 9gm carbs).	

Day 5

1 serving of Pumpkin Bread + 1 tbsp. Cream Cheese – Breakfast (265.8Kcal, 23gm fat, 8.9gm proteins & 4.8gm carbs)

1 serving of Cabbage Slaw + 1 serving of Roasted Zucchini 2 tbsp. Flax Seeds – Lunch (130Kcal, 10gm fat, 2.3gm proteins & 5.1gm carbs)

1 serving of Stuffed Mushrooms + 1 serving of Roasted Broccoli – Dinner (144Kcal, 9.5gm fat, 8gm proteins & 6.3gm carbs)

Chocolate Coconut Balls – Dessert (134Kcal, 7gm fat, 2gm proteins & 21gm carbs).

Day 6

3 serving of Cloud Bread + 3 tbsp. Butter – Breakfast (408kcal, 39gm fat, 2.36gm proteins & 1.3gm carbs)

1 serving of Thai Tofu Curry + 1 serving of Cauliflower Rice – Lunch (345Kcal, 28gm fat, 14gm proteins & 12gm carbs)

1serving of Black Bean Soup – Dinner (296Kcal, 9gm fat, 19gm proteins & 23gm carbs)

Strawberry Smoothie – Dessert (167Kcal, 6gm fat, 16gm proteins & 11gm carbs).

Day 7
1 serving of Berry Mint Smoothie + 5 tbsp. Mixed Nuts – Breakfast (407Kcal, 25gm Fat, 9.4gm proteins & 14gm carbs)
1 serving of Creamed Spinach + 1 serving of Oven Roasted Vegetables – Lunch (425Kcal, 33gm fat, 6gm proteins & 23gm carbs)
1 serving of Greek Broccoli Salad + 1 serving of Grilled Vegetables – Dinner (357Kcal, 25.6gm fat, 12gm proteins & 17gm carbs)
1 serving of Chocolate Fudge – Dessert (154.77Kcal, 15.5gm fat, 7.7gm proteins & 10.79gm carbs).

CHAPTER 3

3.1. BREAKFAST RECIPES

EGG CUPS

Keto & Less than 30 Minutes

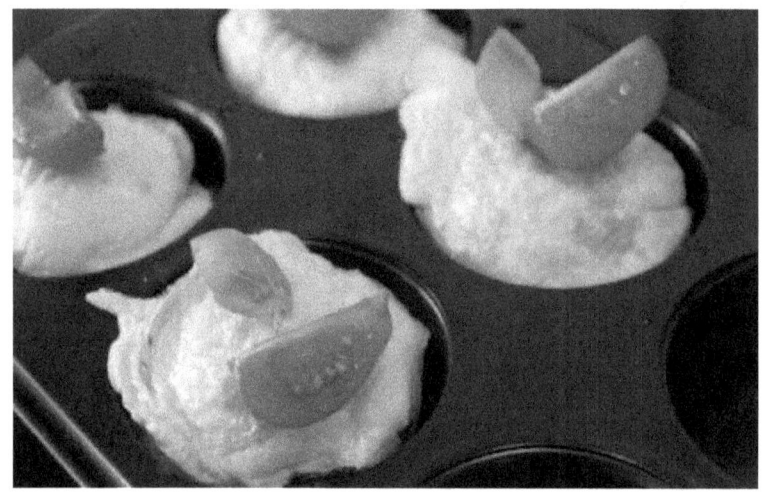

Preparation Time: 5 Minutes

Cooking Time: 15 Minutes

Efforts: Easy

Servings: 12

Nutritional Information per serving:
Calories: 137Kcal, Carbohydrates: 1g, Proteins: 6g,

Fat: 54g, Sodium: 190mg

Ingredients:
- 10 Eggs, large
- ½ tsp. Black Pepper
- 1 ½ tsp. Salt
- ¾ tsp. Italian Seasoning
- ¾ cup Parmesan Cheese, grated
- ½ tsp. Garlic Powder
- 1 cup Spinach, chopped
- 1 cup Tomatoes, ripe & chopped
- ¾ cup Ham, cooked & chopped, optional

Instructions:
1. Preheat the oven to 400° F.
2. Crack the eggs into a large mixing bowl and spoon in salt and pepper.
3. Whisk the mixture well with a whisker.
4. Once combined, stir in garlic powder and Italian seasoning. Mix well and then add spinach, tomato, and cheese. Use ham if needed. Combine.
5. Pour the mixture to greased muffin pans lined with silicone liners.
6. Fill 2/3rd of the cups and add more cheese if desired.
7. Finally, bake them for 13 to 15 minutes or until set.
8. Serve and enjoy.

Tip: Instead of spinach, tomato, and cheese, you can also use broccoli and cheddar cheese combination.

CLOUD BREAD

Keto, GF, Grain-Free & less than 30 minutes

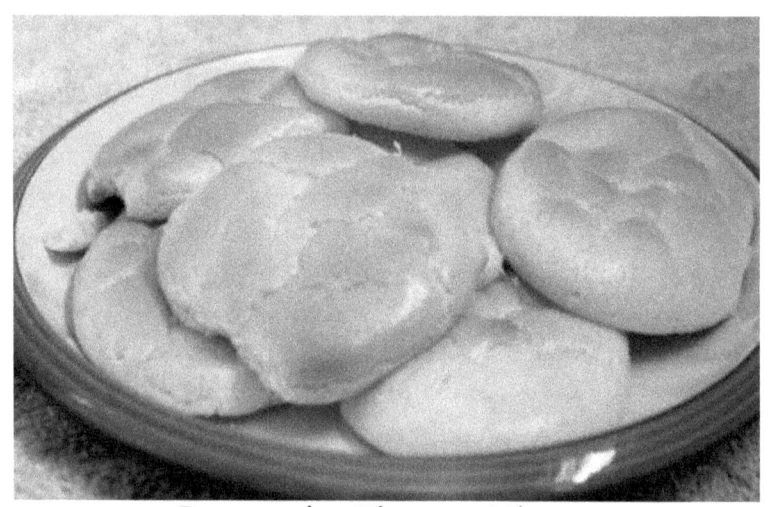

Preparation Time: 10 Minutes

Cooking Time: 15 Minutes

Efforts: Moderate

Servings: 10

Nutritional Information per serving:

Calories: 36Kcal, Carbohydrates: 1g, Proteins: 2g, Fat: 2g, Sodium: 167mg

Ingredients:

- 4 Eggs, large & separated
- ½ tsp. Garlic Powder
- ½ tsp. Cream of Tartar
- ½ tsp. Sea Salt
- 2 oz. Cream Cheese, low-fat
- 1 tsp. Italian Seasoning

Instructions:

1. Preheat the oven to 300° F.
2. Next, keep the egg whites in a large mixing bowl and to this, spoon in the cream of tartar.
3. Whip it on high power until it turns to soft meringue peaks. Transfer to another bowl.
4. Place the cream of cheese into the large bowl and whip on high power to soften.
5. Stir in the egg one by one into the mixture and whisk it well each time before adding each egg. Repeat the procedure until the whole mixture becomes smooth.
6. Spoon in the Italian seasoning, salt, and garlic powder.
7. Gently fold the egg white to the mixture while maintaining the foamy texture.
8. Take ¼ cup portion of the mixture to the greased baking sheet and spread to 4-inch circles. Leave ample space between each.
9. Finally, bake them for 15 to 20 minutes or until they golden on the outside and firm inside.
10. Cool for several minutes and then serve.

Tip: You can reduce the amount of garlic powder if desired.

CREAM CHEESE PANCAKES

Less than 5 ingredients, under 30 Minutes,

Gluten-free & Nut-Free

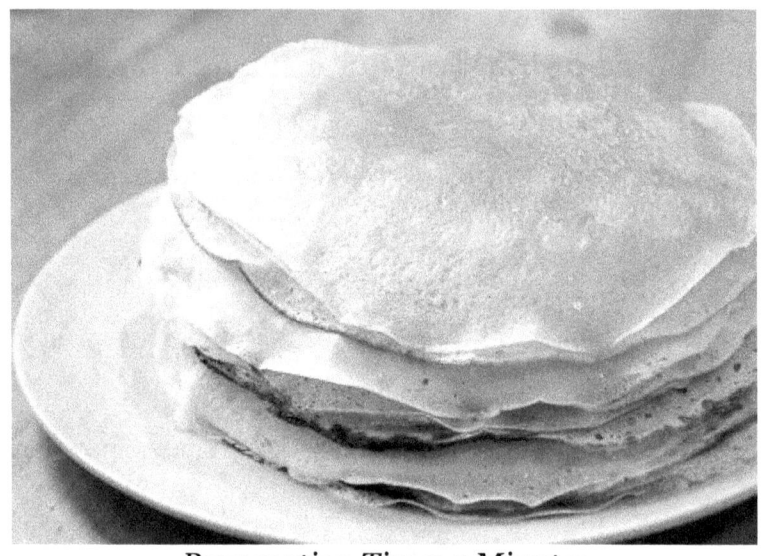

Preparation Time: 5 Minutes

Cooking Time: 10 Minutes

Efforts: Easy

Servings: 1

Nutritional Information per serving:
Calories: 344Kcal, Carbohydrates: 3g, Proteins: 17g,

Fat: 29g, Sodium: 10mg

Ingredients:

- ½ tsp. Cinnamon
- 2 oz. Cream Cheese
- 1 tsp. Low-carb Sweetener, granulated
- 2 Eggs, large

Instructions:

1. Place eggs, cream cheese, sweetener, and cinnamon in a high-speed blender and blend until combined well. Set it aside for 2 minutes.
2. Heat a large-sized skillet over medium heat.
3. When the skillet becomes hot, spoon ¼ of the batter to it and spread it to a circle.
4. Cook for 2 to 3 minutes each side or until cooked. Flip it. Cook the other side for 1 minute.
5. Repeat with the remaining batter and serve.

Tip: Serve it along with sugar-free syrup or berries.

BAGELS

Veg & Less than 5 Ingredient

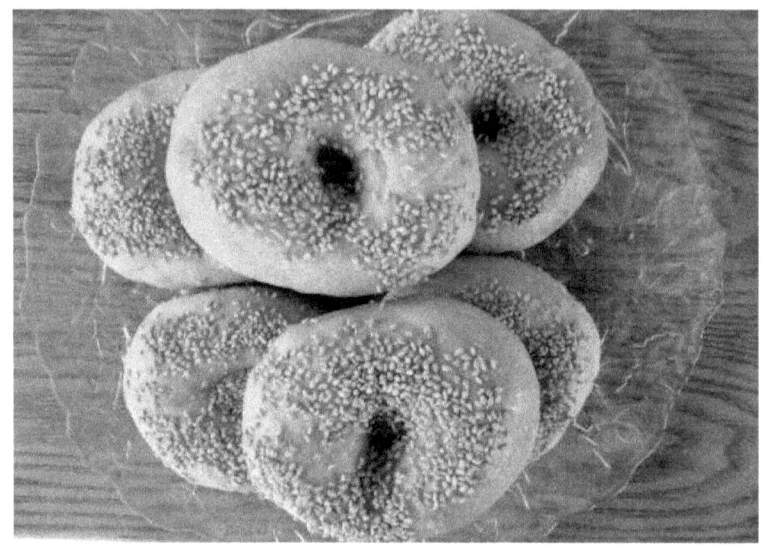

Preparation Time: 15 Minutes

Cooking Time: 15 Minutes

Efforts: Moderate

Servings: 6

Nutritional Information per serving:
Calories: 360Kcal, Carbohydrates: 5g, Proteins: 21g,

Fat: 28g, Sodium: 54mg

Ingredients:
- 1 tbsp. Baking Powder
- 1 ½ cup Almond Flour, blanched
- 2 Eggs, large & beaten

- 2 ½ cup Mozzarella Cheese, shredded
- 2 oz. Cream Cheese, cubed

Instructions:

1. Preheat the oven to 400° F.
2. Combine almond flour and baking powder in a mixing bowl. Set aside.
3. Mix the mozzarella cheese and cream cheese in a large microwave-safe bowl and heat it for 2 minutes on high power. Stir halfway through and at the end.
4. Add the flour mixture and eggs to the cheese mixture and make a dough out of it by kneading it quickly.
5. As the dough will be sticky, keep kneading it until it becomes smooth. Tip: If the dough seems too difficult to mix or is still sticky, you can microwave it again for another 15 to 20 seconds to make it soften.
6. Divide the dough into six portions and roll it into a long log.
7. Press the ends together of the long log to get the bagel shape. Arrange them on a parchment paper-lined baking sheet.
8. Finally, bake them for 12 to 14 minutes or until the bagels are firm and golden in colour.

Tip: You can top it with sesame seeds if desired.

GRANOLA BARS

Veg Keto, under 30 Minutes & Diary-Free

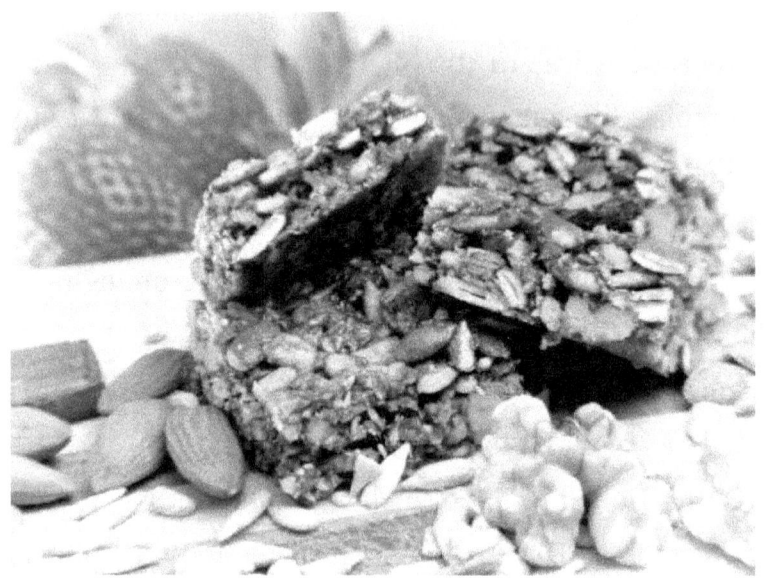

Preparation Time: 10 Minutes

Cooking Time: 15 Minutes

Efforts: Easy

Servings: 12

Nutritional Information per serving:
Calories: 278Kcal, Carbohydrates: 2g, Proteins: 7g,

Fat: 26g, Sodium: 27mg

Ingredients:
- 1 cup Pecans
- 1 cup Almonds
- 1/3 cup Sunflower Seeds
- ½ cup Golden Flaxseed Meal

- 1 cup Hazelnuts
- ¼ cup Butter, melted
- 6 tbsp. Erythritol
- 1 Egg White, large
- 1/3 cup Pumpkin Seeds
- 1 tsp. Vanilla Extract

Instructions:

1. Preheat the oven to 325° F.
2. Place hazelnuts and almonds in a food processor and process until the nuts get chopped.
3. Stir in the pecans and pulse again.
4. Add the pumpkin seeds, sunflower seeds, golden flaxseed, and erythritol to it. Pulse until everything mixes up. Tip: Don't over-process.
5. Pour the egg white to the processor. Mix the vanilla extract and butter in another bowl. Stir again.
6. Pulse a few times again and mix a little of the mixture from the bottom using a spatula. Pulse again until everything coats well. Everything should be a bit damp from the egg white mixture.
7. Transfer the mixture to a parchment paper-lined baking sheet and spread it across evenly.
8. Bake for 18 minutes or until browned slightly at the sides.
9. Cool completely before serving.

Tip: You can spoon a bit of salt if preferred.

PANCAKES

Under 30 Minutes, Veg, Paleo & Diary-Free

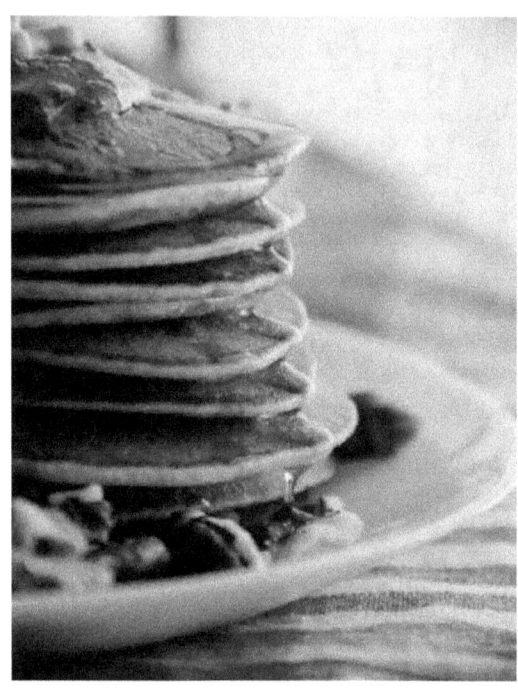

Preparation Time: 5 Minutes

Cooking Time: 15 Minutes

Efforts: Easy

Servings: 6

Nutritional Information per serving:
Calories: 268Kcal, Carbohydrates: 3g, Proteins: 9g,

Fat: 23g, Sodium: 15mg

Ingredients:
- ¼ cup Coconut Flour
- 1 cup Almond Flour, blanched
- 8 tbsp. Almond Milk, unsweetened
- 2 tbsp. Erythritol
- 1 ½ tsp. Vanilla Extract
- 1 tsp. Baking Powder
- 6 Eggs, large

Instructions:

1. Place all the ingredients in a large mixing bowl until combined well.
2. Heat a medium-sized pan over medium-low heat.
3. Pat the pan with ghee and ladle a spoon of batter into the hot pan.
4. Form into circles and cover the pan.
5. Cook for a few minutes or until the bubbles start to appear.
6. Turn the pancake over and cook the other side or until slightly browned.
7. Serve and enjoy.

Tip: You can spoon a bit of salt if preferred.

WAFFLES

Under 30 Minutes, Paleo

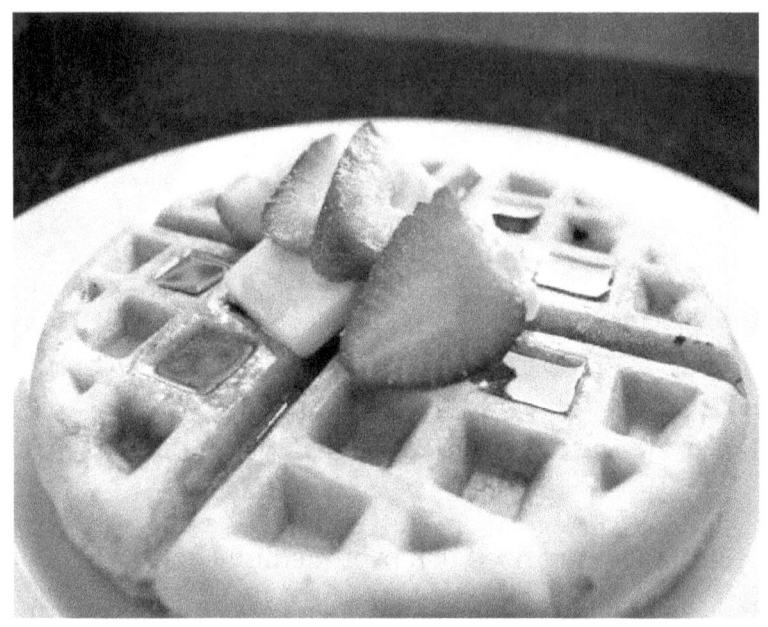

Preparation Time: 10 Minutes

Cooking Time: 10 Minutes

Efforts: Easy

Servings: 2

Nutritional Information per serving:
Calories: 401Kcal, Carbohydrates: 4g, Proteins: 13g,

Fat: 37g, Sodium: 43mg

Ingredients:
- ½ cup Almond Flour, blanched
- ¼ cup Almond Milk, unsweetened
- 1 Egg, large & separated

- 2 tbsp. Butter
- 2 tbsp. Erythritol
- ½ tsp. Vanilla Extract
- ½ tsp. Baking Powder
- 2 tbsp. Nut Butter of your choice
- ¼ tsp. Sea Salt

Instructions:
1. Preheat the waffle iron to high heat and grease it with oil.
2. Crack the egg into a bowl and whisk it until you get stiff peaks.
3. Mix almond flour, salt, erythritol, and baking powder in another bowl. Keep aside.
4. Melt butter and nut butter in a microwave-safe bowl.
5. Spoon this butter mixture to the flour mixture. Combine.
6. Once combined, stir in egg yolk, vanilla essence and almond milk to it and give everything a good stir until you get a smooth mixture.
7. Fold the egg whites gently to the batter so that you get a fluffy and light mixture.
8. Pour half the batter to the waffle iron and close. Cook for 5 minutes or until the steam stops coming. Repeat with the remaining batter.
9. Serve and enjoy.

Tip: For a crispier waffle, you can toast it oven or toaster for a few minutes.

BLUEBERRY MUFFINS

Under 30 Minutes, Paleo & Diary-Free

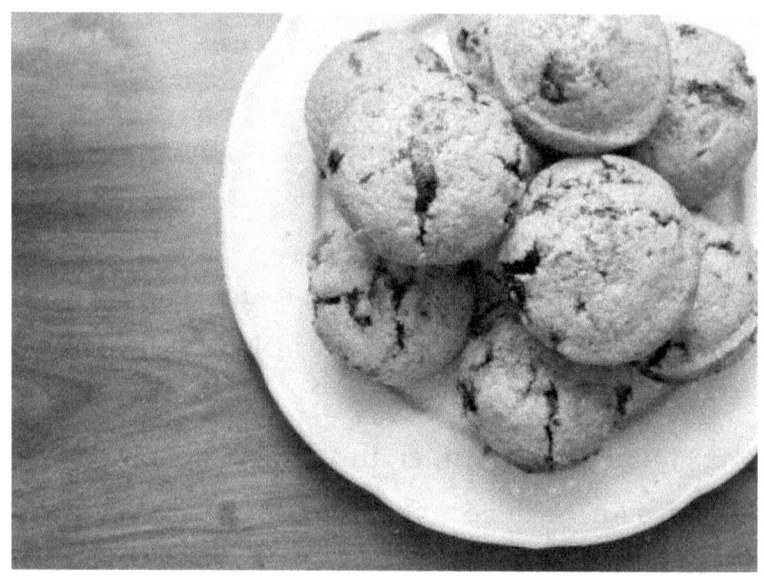

Preparation Time: 10 Minutes

Cooking Time: 20 Minutes

Efforts: Easy

Servings: 12

Nutritional Information per serving:
Calories: 217Kcal, Carbohydrates: 3g, Proteins: 7g,

Fat: 19g, Sodium: 35mg

Ingredients:

- 1 ½ tsp. Baking Powder
- 2 ½ cup Almond Flour, blanched
- 1/3 cup Almond Milk, unsweetened
- ¾ cup Blueberries
- ½ cup Erythritol
- ½ tsp. Vanilla Extract
- 1/3 cup Coconut Oil
- 3 Eggs, large

Instructions:

1. Preheat the oven to 350° F.
2. Combine almond flour, baking powder, salt, and erythritol in a large mixing bowl until mixed well.
3. To this, spoon in the coconut oil, eggs, almond milk, and vanilla extract. Give everything a good stir.
4. Fold in gently the blueberries to the batter.
5. Transfer the mixture to silicone paper muffin liners lined muffin pan and spread across evenly.
6. Bake them for 20 to 25 minutes or until a toothpick inserted in the center comes clean, and the muffin is golden coloured.
7. Serve and enjoy.

Tip: You can add ¼ tsp. of sea salt if desired.

ALMOND FLOUR PORRIDGE

Vegan, Less than 30 Minutes & Paleo

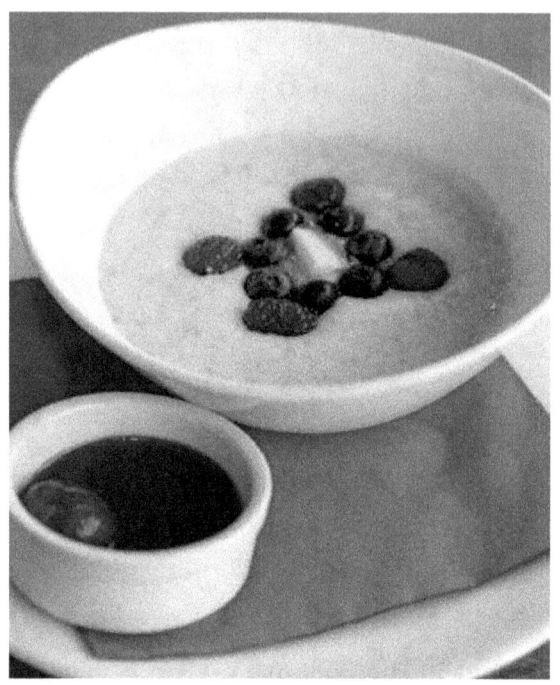

Preparation Time: 5 Minutes

Cooking Time: 5 Minutes

Efforts: Easy

Servings: 1

Nutritional Information per serving:
Calories: 216Kcal, Carbohydrates: 2.5g, Proteins: 8.1g, Fat: 17.4g, Sodium: 5mg

Ingredients:

- 1 tsp. Erythritol, granulated
- 2 tbsp. Flaxseed, grounded
- ½ cup Almond Milk, unsweetened
- 2 tbsp. Almond Flour
- 2 tbsp. Sesame Seeds, grounded

Instructions:

1. Combine the sesame seeds, flaxseed meal, and almond flour in a microwave-safe bowl and mix well.
2. To this, pour the almond milk and heat it on high power for one minute in the microwave.
3. Stir in the mixture and heat it again for one minute. Add more milk if the mixture seems thicker.
4. Sprinkle the erythritol over it and combine it.

Tip: You can top it with berries if desired.

PUMPKIN PANCAKES F

Keto, Dairy-Free & Nut-Free

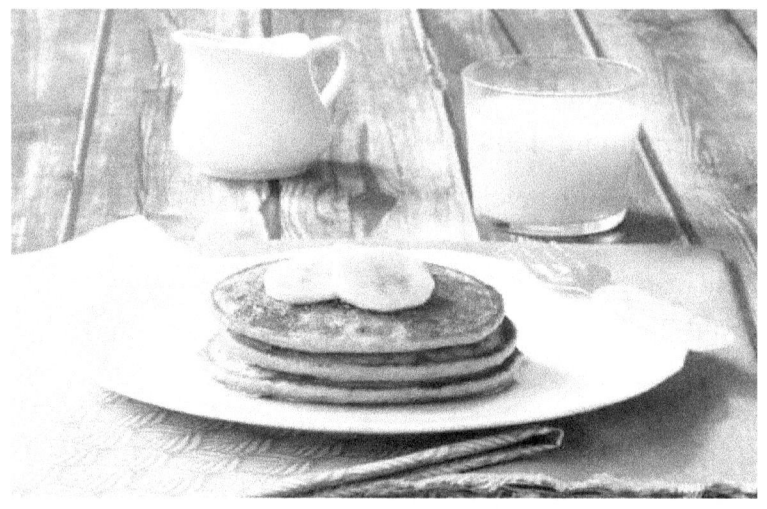

Preparation Time: 10 Minutes

Cooking Time: 20 Minutes

Efforts: Easy

Servings: 16

Nutritional Information per serving:
Calories: 221Kcal, Carbohydrates: 4.2g, Proteins: 10.8g, Fat: 15.4g, Sodium: 13mg

Ingredients:
- ½ cup Pumpkin Puree
- ½ tsp. Vanilla Extract
- ½ cup Coconut Flour
- 3 tbsp. Coconut Oil
- ¼ cup Protein Powder

- ¾ cup Almond Milk, unsweetened
- ¼ cup Swerve Sweetener
- 6 Eggs, large
- 1 tsp. Baking Powder
- ¼ tsp. Cloves
- ½ tsp. Salt
- ½ tsp. Ginger
- 1 tsp. Cinnamon

Instructions:

1. Combine coconut flour, sweetener, cloves, protein powder, ginger, baking powder, salt, and cinnamon in a large mixing bowl.
2. Stir in the eggs, ½ cup almond milk, pumpkin puree, vanilla extract, and coconut oil to it. Mix well.
3. Heat a large pan over medium-high heat, and once it becomes hot, spoon in coconut oil.
4. Pour a ladle of the batter to the skillet and spread it to a circle.
5. Cook them for 4 minutes per side or until it is golden brown.
6. Turn them over and cook the other side.
7. Repeat with the remaining batter.
8. Serve and enjoy it.

Tip: You can top it with more butter.

BANANA BREAD

Gluten Free & Grain Free

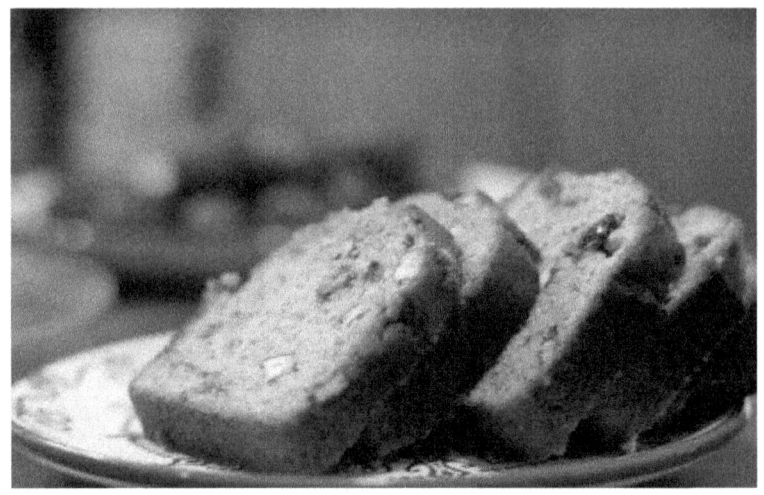

Preparation Time: 10 Minutes

Cooking Time: 40 Minutes

Efforts: Easy

Servings: 8

Nutritional Information per serving:

Calories: 205Kcal, Carbohydrates: 4.4g, Proteins: 8g, Fat: 17.2g, Sodium: 110mg

Ingredients:
- 1 ½ cup Almond Flour
- 2 tsp. Cinnamon
- 3 Eggs, large
- 2 Bananas, small & mashed
- 2 tbsp. Butter
- 1 tsp. Baking Powder
- ¼ cup Erythritol, grounded

Instructions:
1. Preheat the oven to 356° F.
2. Whisk the eggs along with the mashed banana and melted butter until mixed well.
3. Combine the erythritol, baking powder, almond flour, and cinnamon in another bowl.
4. Add the almond flour mixture to the egg-banana mix and give everything a good stir.
5. Transfer the mixture to a greased parchment paper-lined loaf pan.
6. Bake it for 35 to 40 minutes or until a toothpick inserted in the center comes clean. Tip: Check the bread at 30 minutes, and if it already browned but not cooked, then cover it with aluminum foil.

Tip: You can add crushed walnuts if desired for crunchiness.

LOW-CARB BREAD

Paleo & Gluten-Free

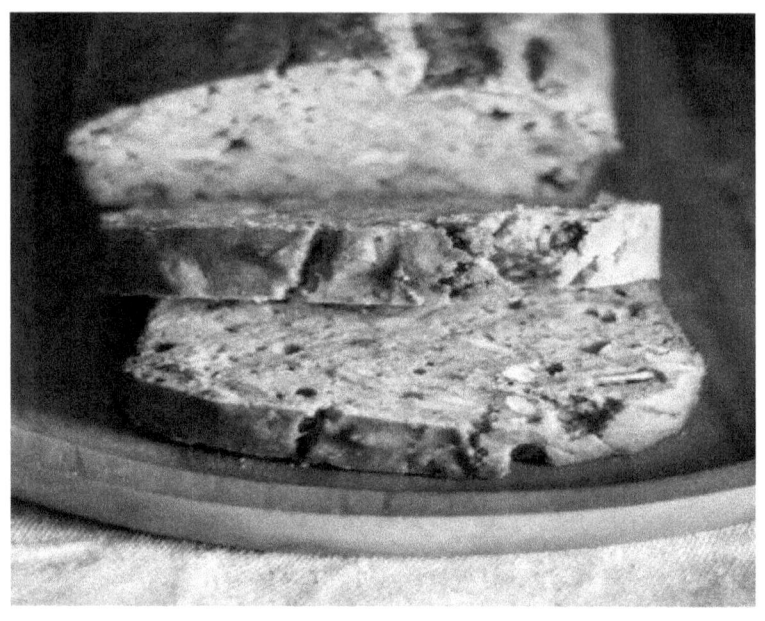

Preparation Time: 10 Minutes

Cooking Time: 30 Minutes

Efforts: Easy

Servings: 4

Nutritional Information per serving:
Calories: 294 Kcal, Carbohydrates: 3g, Proteins: 14g, Fat: 24g, Sodium: 17mg

Ingredients:
- 1/3 cup Oil
- 6 Eggs, separated
- 1 tbsp. Baking Powder
- 2 Eggs, whole
- 2 cups Almond Flour

- ¼ tsp. Cream of Tartar
- Salt, to taste
- Chopped Nuts or Seeds, optional

Instructions:
1. Preheat the oven to 400° F.
2. Separate the eggs yolk and egg white in two separate bowls.
3. Add the two whole egg yolks to it and spoon in the oil.
4. Whisk the mixture until smooth.
5. Stir in the almond flour, a dash of salt and baking powder into it and mix well.
6. Spoon the whole mixture with a spatula until mixed well and keep aside.
7. Spoon in the cream of tartar along with the egg whites in another bowl and beat it with a hand mixer until stiff peaks form.
8. With the spatula, transfer 1/3 of the egg whites mixture to the almond flour mixture. Gently fold the whole batter together.
9. Once combined, add the next 1/3rd of the mixture to the batter and fold in gently.
10. Stir in the remaining egg white until the batter is smooth without any egg white lumps.
11. Pour the mixture to a greased parchment paper-lined loaf pan and bake for 40 minutes or until set.
12. Set aside the bread to cool for 10 minutes and then remove it from the pan. Slice after another 1 hour.
13. Serve and enjoy.

Tip: You can add seeds of your choice if desired.

VEGETABLE FRITTATA

Veg & Under 30 Minutes

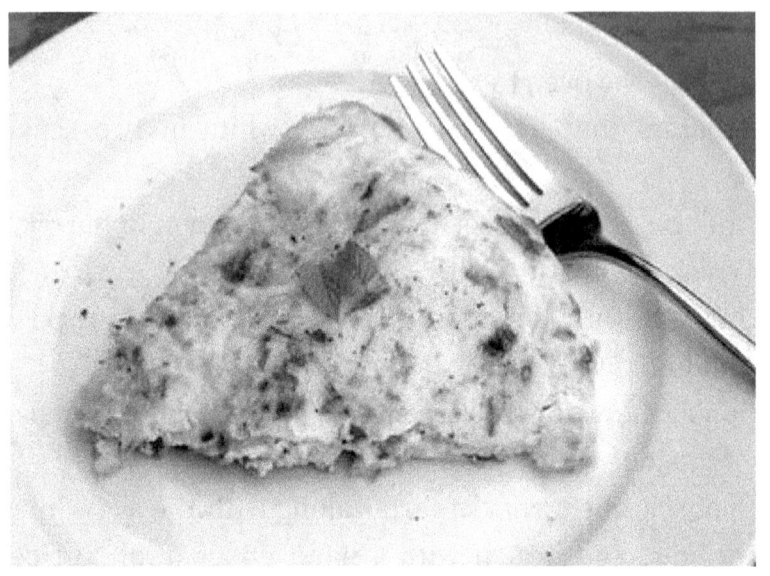

Preparation Time: 10 Minutes

Cooking Time: 20 Minutes

Efforts: Easy

Servings: 4

Nutritional Information per serving:
Calories: 188Kcal, Carbohydrates: 1g, Proteins: 11g,

Fat: 15g, Sodium: 223g

Ingredients:
- 8 Eggs, large
- 2 tbsp. Olive Oil
- 2/3 cup Cheddar Cheese
- 1 ½ cup Mushrooms, sliced
- ¼ tsp. Salt
- 1 cup Bell Peppers, sliced into strips
- ¼ tsp. Black Pepper
- 1 cup Zucchini, sliced into quartered
- ¼ cup Heavy Cream

Instructions:
1. Preheat the oven to 350° F.
2. Spoon oil to a heated cast-iron skillet over medium heat.
3. Stir in the vegetables and cook them for 4 to 6 minutes or until softened.
4. In the meantime, whisk eggs, salt, heavy cream, and pepper in a medium-sized bowl until combined well.
5. Add the egg mixture over the vegetables and add the cheese over it. Mix gently.
6. Transfer the cast-iron skillet to the oven and bake for 18 to 20 minutes or until the top is puffy while being just set in the middle.
7. Allow it to cool for 10 minutes before serving.

Tip: You can add your choice of low-carb veggies to it.

PUMPKIN BREAD

Paleo, Dairy-Free & Keto

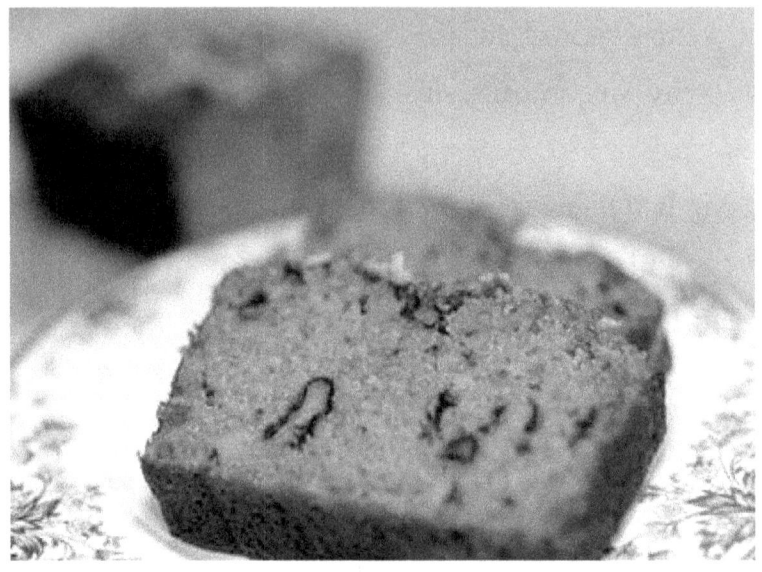

Preparation Time: 10 Minutes

Cooking Time: 50 Minutes

Efforts: Easy

Servings: 12

Nutritional Information per serving:
Calories: 215Kcal, Carbohydrates: 4g, Proteins: 8g,

Fat: 18g, Sodium: 147g

Ingredients:
- ¾ cup Pumpkin Puree
- ¼ cup Pumpkin Seeds
- 2 cups Almond Flour, blanched
- 1/3 cup Butter
- ½ cup Coconut Flour
- 4 Eggs, large
- ¾ cup Erythritol
- ¼ tsp. Sea Salt
- 2 tsp. Baking Powder
- 2 tsp. Pumpkin Spice

Instructions:
1. Preheat the oven to 350° F.
2. Mix all the dry ingredients in a large mixing bowl until combined well.
3. In another bowl, beat together eggs, pumpkin puree and melted butter with a whisker until combined.
4. Transfer the batter to a parchment paper-lined so that the paper hangs over the sides. Smoothen the top and garnish it with pumpkin seeds.
5. Bake for 55 to 60 minutes or until a toothpick inserted in the center comes clean.
6. Allow it to cool for some time before slicing.

Tip: Serve it along with cream cheese.

KETO SCRAMBLED EGGS

Keto, Under 30 Minutes

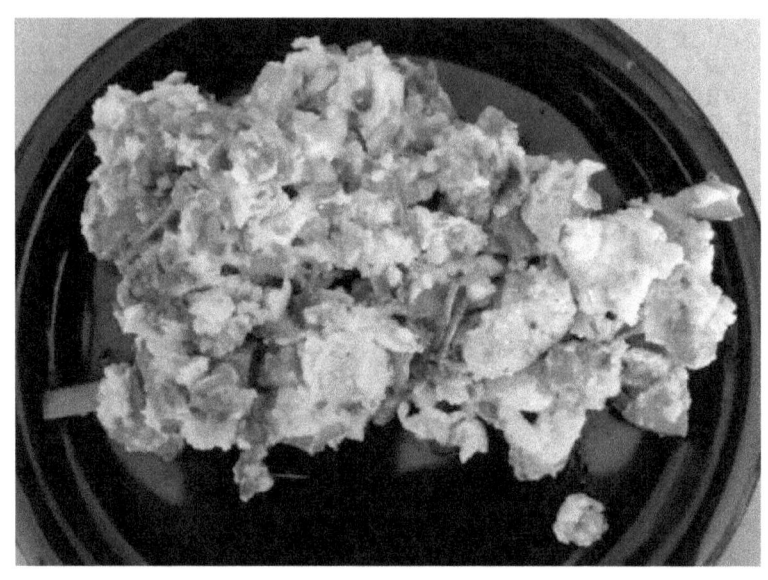

Preparation Time: 10 Minutes

Cooking Time: 20 Minutes

Efforts: Easy

Servings: 2

Nutritional Information per serving:
Calories: 455Kcal, Carbohydrates: 4g, Proteins: 14g, Fat: 43g, Sodium: 641g

Ingredients:
- 4 Eggs, large
- 2 tbsp. Scallions, sliced thinly
- 3 tbsp. Butter
- ½ tsp. Salt
- 1/3 cup Heavy Cream
- 2 tbsp. Cilantro, chopped
- 1 Serrano Chili Pepper
- Dash of Pepper
- 1 Tomato, small & chopped

Instructions:

1. Melt the butter by heating a large non-stick pan over medium-high heat.
2. Once the pan is hot, stir in the chili and tomato to it and cook for 2 minutes.
3. Mix eggs, pepper, cream, salt, and chili in a medium bowl with a whisker until combined well.
4. Pour the egg mixture to the pan and allow it to cook.
5. With a spatula, fold the edges toward the center. Tip: Allow the egg to set around the edges.
6. Continue cooking for a few more minutes or until soft.
7. Serve it hot.

Tip: You can add more low-carb veggies if preferred.

AVOCADO TOAST

Less than 5 ingredients,

Under 30 Minutes & Veg

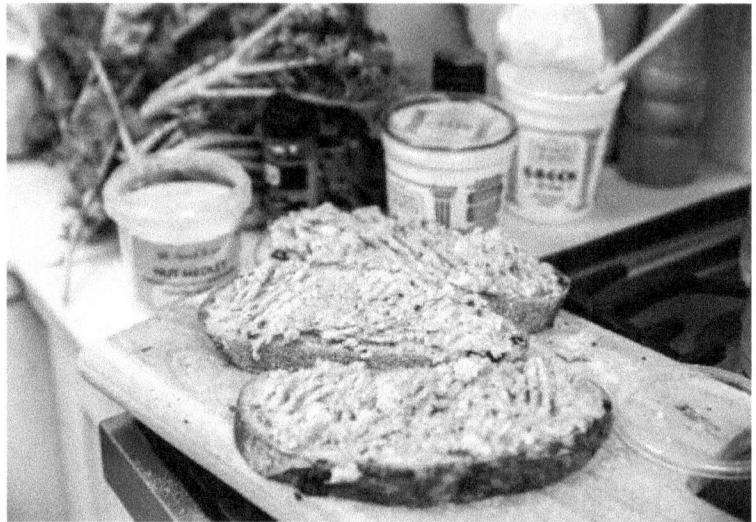

Preparation Time: 10 Minutes

Cooking Time: 15 Minutes

Efforts: Easy

Servings: 1

Nutritional Information per serving:

Calories: 460Kcal, Carbohydrates: 2.1g, Proteins: 17.5g,

Fat: 37.4g, Sodium: 471g

Ingredients:
- 2 Slices of Low-Carb Bread
- ½ of 1 Avocado, sliced or mashed
- Dash of Sea Salt
- ½ to ¾ tsp. Olive Oil
- Pinch of Red Pepper Flakes

Instructions:
1. Heat a cast-iron skillet over medium heat.
2. Once it is heated, place the bread slice over it and cook for one minute or until toasted.
3. Remove the bread from the skillet and top it with sliced or mashed avocado and seasonings.
4. Serve and enjoy it.

Tip: You can add bacon and cheese if desired.

CAULIFLOWER HASH

BrownsLess than 5 ingredients, Diary-Free & Keto

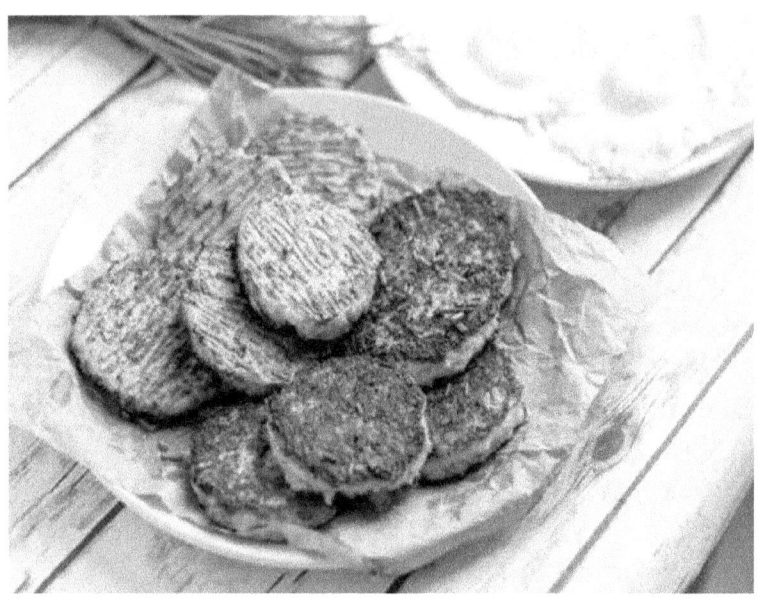

Preparation Time: 10 Minutes

Cooking Time: 30 Minutes

Efforts: Easy

Servings: 4

Nutritional Information per serving:
Calories: 282Kcal, Carbohydrates: 3g, Proteins: 7g,

Fat: 26g, Sodium: 356g

Ingredients:

- 1 lb. Cauliflower, washed, trimmed & grated
- Salt & Pepper, as needed
- 3 Eggs, medium
- 4 oz. Butter
- ½ of 1 Yellow Onion

Instructions:

1. Place the grated cauliflower in a medium-sized bowl.
2. Add and stir in the remaining ingredients, excluding the butter and mix well.
3. Melt the butter in a large frying pan over medium heat.
4. Once melted, scoop out the cauliflower mixture to the pan and spread them out slightly.
5. Cook them for 4 minutes per side or until cooked. Tip: They might fall apart if taken too soon.

Tip: Serve along with a salad.

BACON & EGGS

Under 30 Minutes, Keto & Less than 5 ingredients

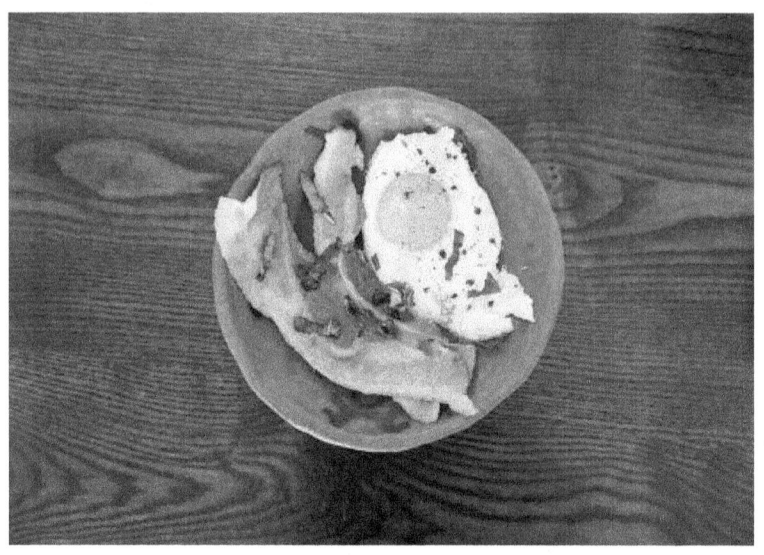

Preparation Time: 5 Minutes

Cooking Time: 20 Minutes

Efforts: Easy

Servings: 2

Nutritional Information per serving:
Calories: 272Kcal, Carbohydrates: 1g, Proteins: 15g,

Fat: 22g, Sodium: 280g

Ingredients:
- 4 Eggs, large
- 2 ½ oz. Bacon, sliced
- Sprigs of Parsley, fresh & chopped

Instructions:
1. Heat a medium-sized pan over high heat, and once it becomes hot, fry the bacon in it until it becomes crispy. Set it aside on a plate and leave the fat in the pan.
2. Crack the eggs into the bacon grease.
3. Cook the eggs according to your preference.
4. Add salt and pepper as needed.
5. Serve it hot and top it with the parsley.

Tip: If preferred, you can even top it with sliced cherry tomatoes.

BUTTER COFFEE

Under 30 Minutes,

Keto & Less than 5 ingredients

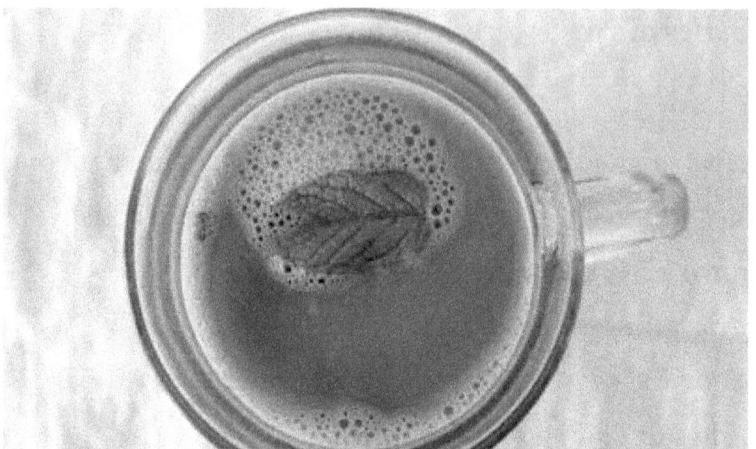

Preparation Time: 5 Minutes

Cooking Time: 1 Minute

Efforts: Easy

Servings: 1

Nutritional Information per serving:
Calories: 334Kcal, Carbohydrates: 0g, Proteins: 1g,

Fat: 38g, Sodium: 27g

Ingredients:
- 1 cup Hot Coffee, freshly brewed
- 1 tbsp. MCT Oil or Coconut Oil
- 2 tbsp. Butter, unsalted

Instructions:
1. Placing the hot coffee, butter, and MCT oil in a blender and blend until frothy.
2. Serve immediately.

Tip: If preferred, you can add cocoa powder or pumpkin spice.

3.2 LUNCH

CHERRY PORK TENDERLOIN

Gluten-Free & Keto

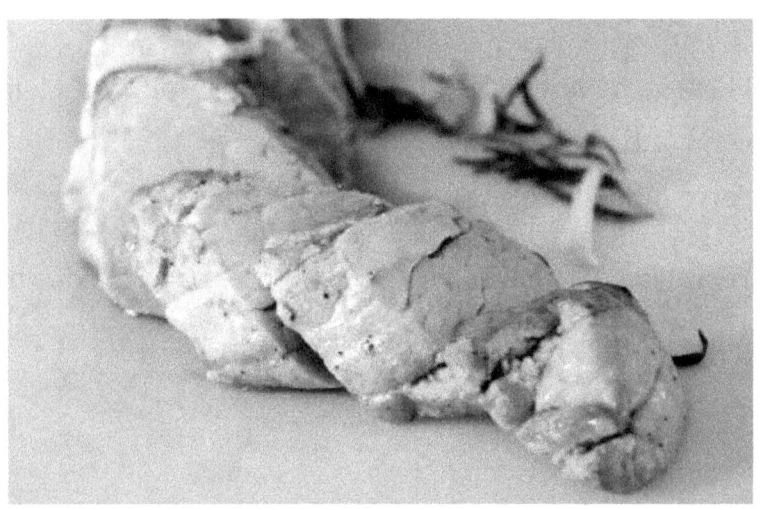

Preparation Time: 10 Minutes

Cooking Time: 15 Minutes + 40 Minutes

Efforts: Easy

Servings: 6

Nutritional Information per serving:
Calories: 330Kcal, Carbohydrates: 10g, Proteins: 36g,

Fat: 16g, Sodium: 490mg

Ingredients:
- 2 Pork Tenderloins, chopped & trimmed of excess fat
- 1 ½ cup Cherries, halved & pitted
- ½ tsp. Black Pepper

- ½ cup Balsamic Vinegar
- 2 cloves of Garlic
- ¼ cup Extra-Virgin Olive Oil
- 1 tsp. Salt
- 1 tbsp. Honey
- 1 tbsp. Dijon Mustard
- 2 tsp. Thyme, fresh

Instructions:

1. Place all the ingredients excluding the pork tenderloin in a high-speed blender and blend for 45 seconds or until it becomes smooth & pureed.
2. Keep the pork in a resealable plastic bag and pour about 1 ¾ cup of the marinade into it. Seal it and shake well so that the meat coats the marinade well.
3. Keep the meat for marination in the refrigerator for at least 30 minutes, or if time permits, you can even keep it for 24 hours.
4. Before grilling, keep the meat outside about 30 minutes before cooking. Heat the grill on medium-high heat.
5. Place the meat onto the center portion of the grill while discarding the marinade.
6. Cook for 11 to 15 minutes while keeping it covered.
7. Turn the pork every 5 minutes or until the meat reaches an internal temperature of 140° F.
8. Take the pork from the grill and allow it to rest for 10 minutes before serving. Serve the remaining marinade ¾ cup of marinade for serving.

Tip: If you prefer, you can even roast the meat in the oven at 400° F for 30 minutes.

TUNA TARTARE

No-cook, Keto & Under 30 Minutes

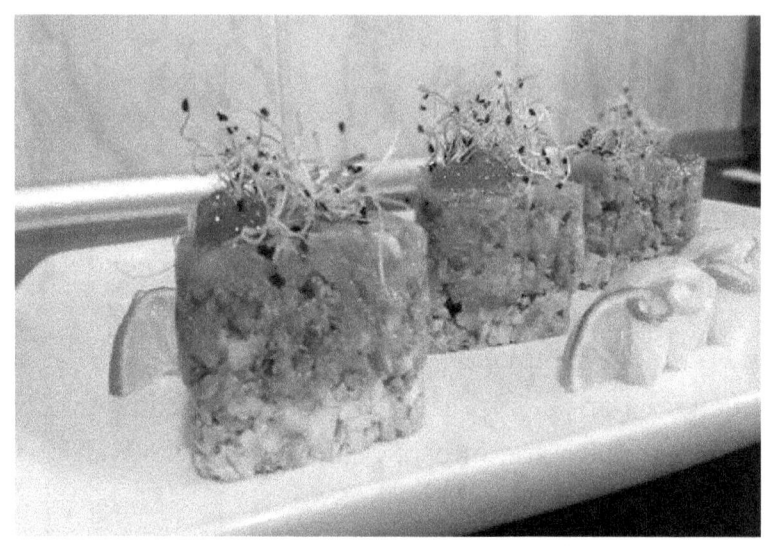

Preparation Time: 30 Minutes

Cooking Time: 0 Minutes

Efforts: Easy

Servings: 4

Nutritional Information per serving:
Calories: 280Kcal, Carbohydrates: 2.6g, Proteins: 27.8g, Fat: 15.6g, Sodium: 211mg

Ingredients:
- 2 tsp. Extra Virgin Olive Oil
- 1 Avocado, diced
- 1 lb. Sushi-grade Tuna

- 2 tsp. Sesame Oil
- 2 tbsp. Chives, fresh & chopped finely
- 2 Persian Cucumber
- Pinch of Cayenne Pepper
- 2 tbsp. Red Onion, chopped finely
- ¼ tsp. Salt
- 2 Crispy Seaweed Sheets, optional

Instructions:

1. Keep the tuna in the freezer for 10 to 20 minutes or until it is firm.
2. Combine sesame oil, salt, chives, cayenne, onion, and olive oil in a medium-sized bowl. Keep it aside.
3. Place the tuna on the cutting board and cut thin slices along the grain with a sharp knife.
4. Slice them lengthwise and turn them. Chop the tuna to diced about 1/8th inch.
5. Transfer the tuna to the mixing bowl and gently mix them with the ingredients. Check for seasoning.
6. For serving, place the cucumber slices and top it with a generous amount of tuna tartare and diced avocado. If using seaweed sheets, garnish with it.

Tip: For more flavor, you can add black finishing salt at the end as a garnish.

GRILLED SALMON

Under 30 Minutes,

Keto & Less than 5-ingredients

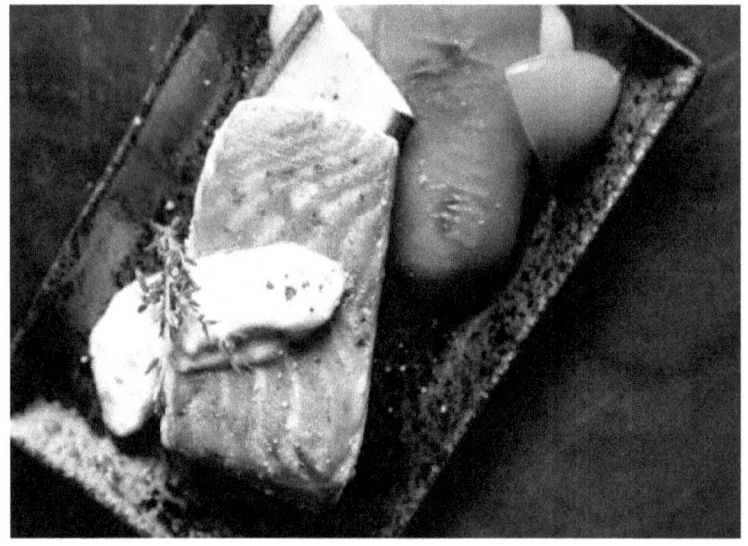

Preparation Time: 10 Minutes

Cooking Time: 10 Minutes

Efforts: Easy

Servings: 2

Nutritional Information per serving:

Calories: 262Kcal, Carbohydrates: 4g, Proteins: 42g,

Fat: 9g, Sodium: 154mg

Ingredients:

- 1 lb. Salmon Fillet, sliced into smaller fillets
- 1 Lemon, large & sliced into rounds
- 1 tbsp. Avocado Oil
- ¼ tsp. Sea Salt
- 1 tbsp. Herbs De Province or Italian Seasoning

Instructions:

1. Preheat the grill to medium-high.
2. Keep the salmon fillets on a large foil sheet.
3. Spoon the avocado oil over it and brush it all over the fillets.
4. Add the Italian seasoning and sea salt over the fillets and coat them over it.
5. Top them with the lemon slices and wrap in aluminum foil to make a foil packet.
6. Place them on the grill and cook them for 10 to 15 minutes or until the fish is cooked while keeping it covered.
7. Remove the fish from the grill and unwrap the foil when it is cool to handle.
8. Serve it hot.

Tip: For more flavor, you can add more herbs.

BROCCOLI BACON SALAD

Keto & Under 30 Minutes

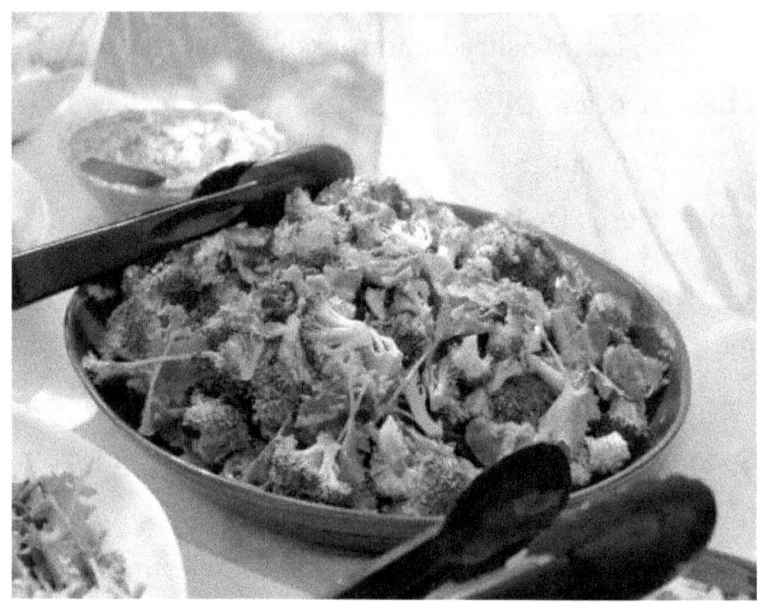

Preparation Time: 10 Minutes

Cooking Time: 10 Minutes

Efforts: Easy

Servings: 8

Nutritional Information per serving:
Calories: 386.7Kcal, Carbohydrates: 8.33g, Proteins: 15.24g, Fat: 30.73g, Sodium: 365mg

Ingredients:

- 6 oz. Bacon, cooked & crumbled
- ½ cup Pumpkin Seeds
- 3 tbsp. Apple Cider Vinegar
- Salt & Pepper, as needed
- ½ of 1 Red Onion, medium & diced
- 5 tbsp. Erythritol
- ¾ cup Mayonnaise, low-carb
- 4 oz. Cheddar Cheese

Instructions:

1. Mix the broccoli, cheddar cheese, red onion, and pumpkin seeds in a large mixing bowl.
2. In another bowl, combine mayonnaise, apple cider vinegar, and erythritol.
3. Spoon the mayonnaise mixture to the broccoli mixture and mix well.
4. Add salt and pepper as needed. Place the mixture in the refrigerator at least for 3 hours for the flavors to meld.
5. Finally, spoon in the crumbled bacon and stir.
6. Serve and enjoy it.

Tip: For more flavor, you can add more herbs like parsley.

CHICKEN SOUP

Keto & Nut-Free

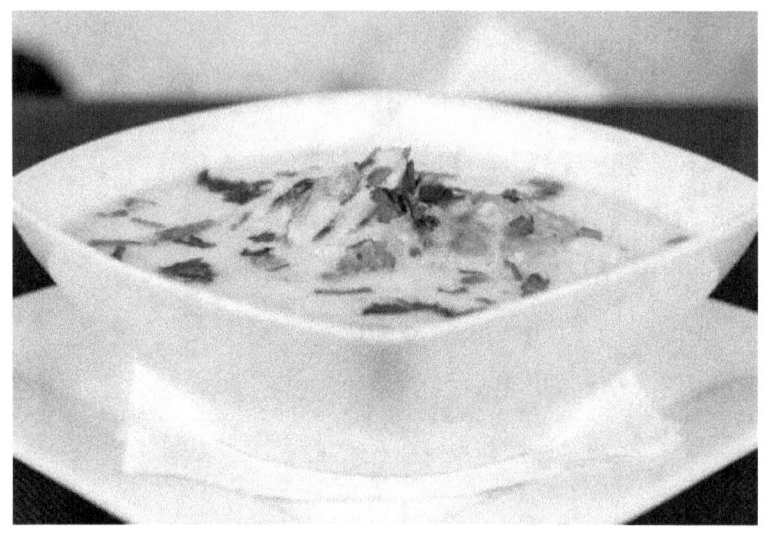

Preparation Time: 10 Minutes

Cooking Time: 20 Minutes

Efforts: Easy

Servings: 6

Nutritional Information per serving:
Calories: 274Kcal, Carbohydrates: 6g, Proteins: 26g,

Fat: 15g, Sodium: 465mg

Ingredients:
- 16 oz. Chicken, cooked & diced
- 6 cups Bone Broth
- 1 Bay Leaf, whole
- ¼ cup White Wine, dry
- 8 oz. Celery Root, cubed

- Salt & Pepper, as needed
- ½ of 1 Onion, diced
- 2 tsp. Chicken Bouillon
- 1/3 cup Carrot, roll cut
- 1 Garlic clove, large & sliced
- 1 tbsp. Garlic Powder
- 4 tbsp. Butter
- 1 cup Celery, sliced
- 1 tsp. Lemon Zest

Instructions:

1. In a pot over medium-high heat add butter.
2. Once the butter has melted, stir in all the vegetables, bay leaf, and lemon zest. Mix well.
3. Lower the heat and spoon in the garlic powder, chicken bouillon, and wine. Combine.
4. Cover the pot and cook for 4 minutes or until the vegetables are sweated bit not browned.
5. Pour the bone broth and bring the mixture to a boil.
6. Lower the heat and allow the mixture to simmer until the vegetables get cooked.
7. When the vegetables become tender, add the chicken, salt, and pepper.
8. Serve it hot.

Tip: Pair it with shirataki noodles or spiralized zucchini.

BEEF STEW

Keto & Diary-Free

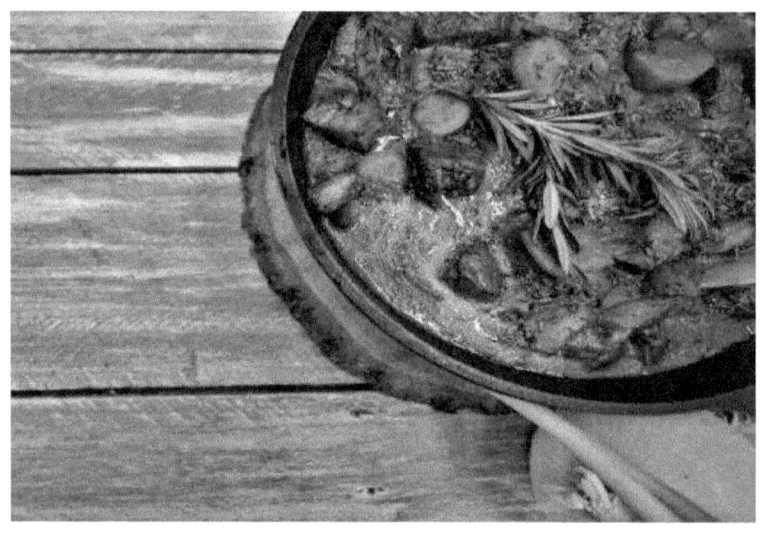

Preparation Time: 20 Minutes

Cooking Time: 2 Hour 10 Minutes

Efforts: Easy

Servings: 6

Nutritional Information per serving:

Calories: 288Kcal, Carbohydrates: 6g, Proteins: 20g,

Fat: 20g, Sodium: 366mg

Ingredients:

- 3 oz. Carrot, roll-cut
- 1 ¼ lb. Chuck Roast Beef, trimmed & cubed into 1-inch
- 2 tbsp. Tomato Paste
- 1 Bay Leaf, large
- 6 oz. Celery Root, peeled & cubed into 3/4th inch
- 2 Garlic cloves, sliced

- 8 oz. Mushroom, whole & quartered
- 3 Celery Ribs, sliced
- 4 oz. Pearl Onions, trimmed & peeled
- ½ tsp. Thyme, dried
- Salt & Pepper, to taste
- 2 tbsp. Olive Oil
- ½ tsp. Thyme, dried
- 5 cups Beef Broth

Instructions:

1. Heat a Dutch oven over medium heat, and once it becomes hot, spoon in the oil.
2. Swirl the oil and then stir in the mushrooms. Cook for 2 minutes and remove them from the pot.
3. Add the beef cubes in batches to the pot along with bay leaf, thyme, tomato paste, and more oil.
4. Mix them well for a minute and pour one cup of the beef broth to it while scraping up the burnt bits from the bottom of the pan.
5. Add the remaining broth and bring the mixture to a boil.
6. Lower the heat and cover the pot. Simmer it for 1 ½ hour.
7. After an 1 ½ hour, check for the doneness of the meat. If the meat is still hard, cook for another 20 minutes.
8. When the meat becomes tender, stir in the vegetables and raise the heat until it simmers.
9. Reduce heat. Simmer uncovered for another 40 minutes or until both the vegetables and meat is tender.
10. Taste for seasoning and spoon in more salt and pepper as needed.
11. Serve and enjoy it.

Tip: For more flavor, add ½ cup of red wine along with tomato paste.

MEATLOAF

Keto & Diary-Free

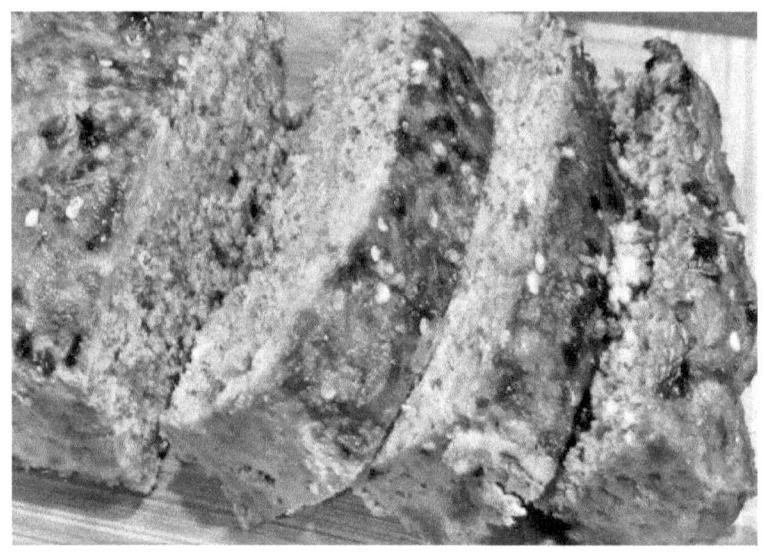

Preparation Time: 10 Minutes

Cooking Time: 45 Minutes

Efforts: Easy

Servings: 4

Nutritional Information per serving:

Calories: 472Kcal, Carbohydrates: 4.25g, Proteins: 15.24g,

Fat: 25g, Sodium: 665mg

Ingredients:

- 2 Eggs
- 1 ½ lb. Beef, grounded
- 4 oz. Tomato Sauce, low-carb
- 1/3 cup Red Onions, chopped
- 1/3 cup Ketchup, keto-approved
- ½ cup Pork Rinds, crushed
- 1 ½ tsp. Chili Powder
- 1/3 tsp. Black Pepper, grounded
- 1 ½ tsp. Mustard, grounded
- 2 tsp. Garlic, minced
- 1 tbsp. Worcestershire Sauce

Instructions:

1. Preheat the oven to 375° F.
2. Mix all the ingredients needed to make the meatloaf excluding the ketchup in a large mixing bowl.
3. Once everything is combined, transfer the mixture to a greased loaf pan and press it down lightly. Smothen the top.
4. Bake the meat mixture for 48 to 50 minutes or until cooked. Allow it to cool for 5 minutes.
5. Spoon the ketchup over the meatloaf and slice it.

Tip: Serve it along with mashed cauliflower.

PULLED PORK

Keto & Diary-Free

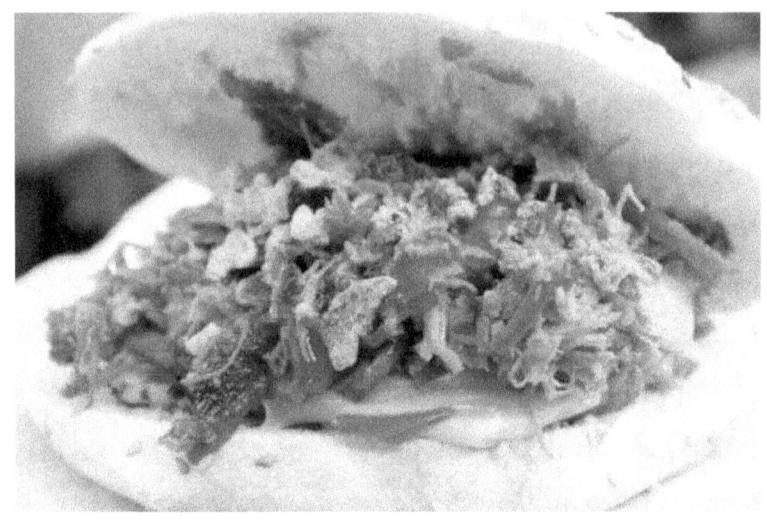

Preparation Time: 10 Minutes

Cooking Time: 2 Hours 10 Minutes

Efforts: Easy

Servings: 10.

Nutritional Information per serving:
Calories: 495Kcal, Carbohydrates: 4g, Proteins: 43g,

Fat: 15g, Sodium: 486mg

Ingredients:
- ¾ cup White Vinegar
- 1 tsp. Mustard, grounded
- 2 Chili Peppers, chopped
- 1 tsp. Salt

- 2 tbsp. Onion, minced
- 1 tsp. Paprika
- 2 tsp. Worcestershire Sauce
- 6 cloves of Garlic, chopped
- 3 tbsp. Tomato Paste
- 4 lb. Pork Butt Shoulder Roast
- 1 Bay Leaf
- 2 tsp. Chili Powder
- ¼ tsp. Low-Carb Sweetener

Instructions:

1. Combine all the ingredients excluding the pork and bay leaf in a large pot until smooth.
2. To this, stir in the pork and coat it with the sauce.
3. Add bay leaf and 1 quart of water into it. Bring the mixture to a boil.
4. Allow the stew to simmer for 1 ½ to 2 hours while keeping the pot covered. Stir frequently.
5. When the pork gets cooked, take the pot from the heat. Keep pork in the sauce until cooled.
6. Once the meat has cooled in the sauce, remove it from the sauce and shred it. Keep aside.
7. Reduce the sauce to 2/3rd and then add the shredded pork.
8. Check for seasoning and add more salt if desired.
9. Serve and enjoy it.

Tip: Serve it as filling for sandwiches or tacos.

CHEESEBURGER SQUASH CASSEROLE

Keto & Nut-Free

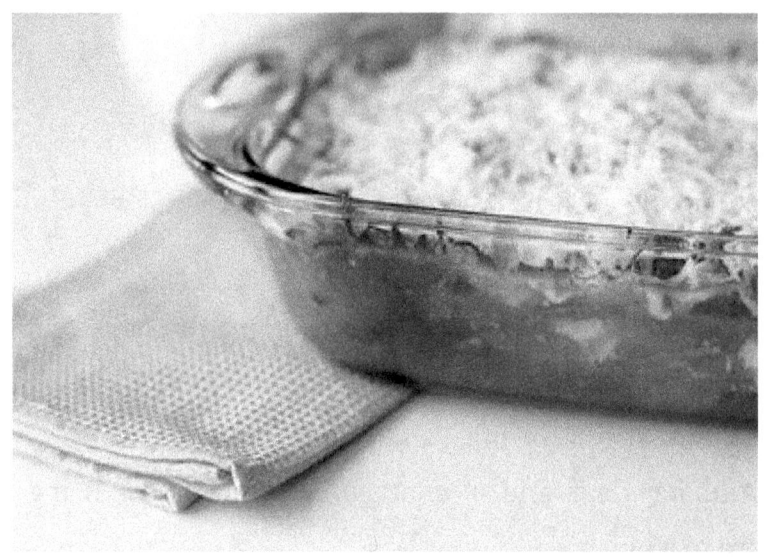

Preparation Time: 10 Minutes

Cooking Time: 1 Hour 15 Minutes

Efforts: Easy

Servings: 6

Nutritional Information per serving:
Calories: 431Kcal, Carbohydrates: 5g, Proteins: 30.5g,

Fat: 28.8g, Sodium: 226mg

Ingredients:
- 6 oz. Cheddar Cheese, shredded
- 1 Squash, medium & sliced into two
- 2 tsp. Worcestershire Sauce

- 4 Bacon Slices, chopped
- 2 tbsp. Ketchup, sugar-free
- 1 lb. Beef, grounded
- ½ Salt & Pepper
- 2 Garlic cloves, minced

Instructions:

1. Preheat the oven to 400° F.
2. Scoop out the seeds and place the squash cut side down. Bake them for 40 minutes or until the squash becomes softened.
3. Meanwhile, cook the bacon in a medium-sized pan over medium heat until crispy.
4. Set the cooked bacon on a paper-towel-lined plate and then place the ground beef in the pan.
5. Cook them for 8 minutes or until browned while stirring them to avoid clumps.
6. Spoon in the garlic, salt, and pepper. Mix.
7. Continue cooking for a few more minutes until the beef until there are no traces of pink colour.
8. Pour the Worcestershire sauce and ketchup into the pan. Scoop out the spaghetti from the squash with a fork.
9. Add the spaghetti to it and mix well with the sauce. Spread out the mixture evenly.
10. Top it with cheese and cover the sauce and meat. Lower the heat and allow the cheese to melt. Cook for 5 minutes.
11. Top it with the bacon and serve.

Tip: Top it with more chopped bacon if desired.

PIMENTO CHEESE BALLS

Under 30 minutes & Keto

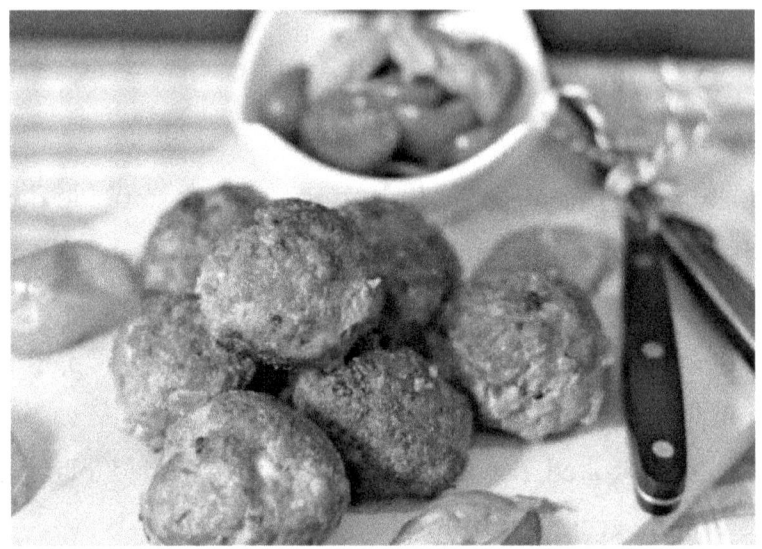

Preparation Time: 10 Minutes

Cooking Time: 10 Minutes

Efforts: Easy

Servings: 4

Nutritional Information per serving:

Calories: 651Kcal, Carbohydrates: 1g, Proteins: 41g,

Fat: 52g, Sodium: 543mg

Ingredients:

For the meatballs:

- 1 ½ lb. Beef, grounded
- 2 tbsp. Butter, for frying
- 1 Egg
- Salt & Pepper, as needed

For the pimiento cheese:

- 1/3 cup Mayonnaise
- Dash of Cayenne Pepper
- 1 tbsp. Dijon Mustard
- ¼ cup Pimentos
- 4 oz. Cheddar Cheese, grated
- 1 tsp. Paprika Powder

Instructions:

1. Place all the ingredients needed to make the pimento cheese in a large mixing bowl.
2. Stir in the beef and egg to the mixture and mix with a spoon until everything comes together.
3. Taste for seasoning and spoon in salt and pepper as needed.
4. Make meatballs out of this meat mixture.
5. Melt the butter in a medium-sized frying pan over medium-high heat.
6. Once the oil is hot, stir in the meatballs and fry them for 2 to 3 minutes or until cooked.
7. Serve it hot.

Tip: Serve it along with green salad and low-carb mayonnaise.

SEAFOOD CHOWDER

Keto & Nuts-Free

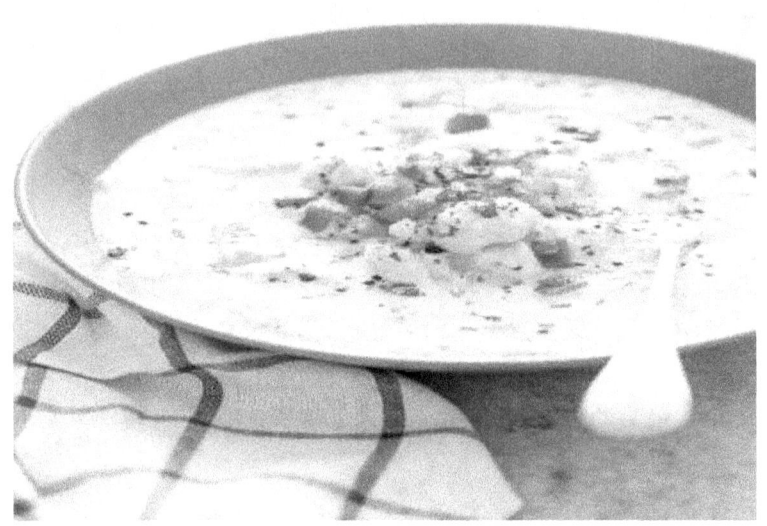

Preparation Time: 20 Minutes

Cooking Time: 20 Minutes

Efforts: Easy

Servings: 4

Nutritional Information per serving:
Calories: 795Kcal, Carbohydrates: 6g, Proteins: 37g,

Fat: 69g, Sodium: 546mg

Ingredients:
- 2 oz. Baby Spinach
- 4 tbsp. Butter
- 2 tsp. Sage, dried

- 2 cloves of Garlic, minced
- 1 lb. Salmon, cut into fillets
- 5 oz. Celery Stalks, sliced
- 2 oz. Baby Spinach
- 1 cup Clam Juice
- 8 oz. Shrimp, peeled & deveined
- 1 ½ cup Heavy Whipping Cream
- ½ tbsp. Red Chili Pepper
- Zest & Juice of ½ of 1 Lemon
- Salt & Pepper, as needed
- 4 oz. Cream Cheese

Instructions:

1. Spoon in butter into a heated large pot over medium heat.
2. Spoon in the garlic and celery. Saute for 5 minutes while stirring it occasionally.
3. Add clam juice, cream cheese, lemon zest, cream, sage, and lemon juice. Mix well.
4. Simmer for about 10 minutes.
5. Stir in the fish and shrimp. Cook for a few minutes or until the fish flakes.
6. Add spinach and cook until wilted.
7. Taste for seasoning and spoon in salt and pepper as needed.
8. Top it with red chili and sage before serving.

Tip: Spoon in red chili pepper flakes for more spiciness.

ZUCCHINI NOODLES WITH PESTO

Veg & Keto

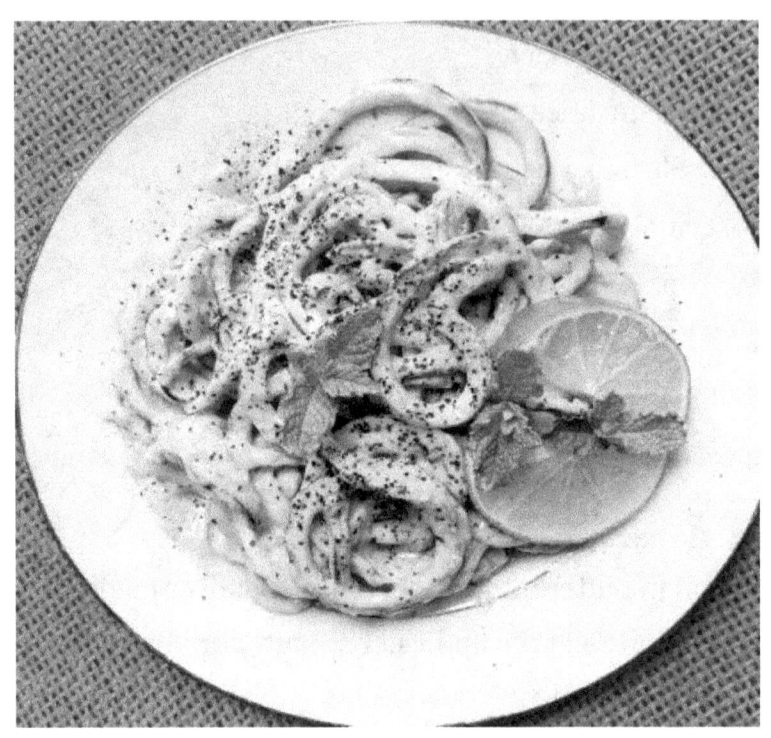

Preparation Time: 15 Minutes

Cooking Time: 15 Minutes

Efforts: Easy

Servings: 4

Nutritional Information per serving:

Calories: 224Kcal, Carbohydrates: 5g, Proteins: 5g,

Fat: 20g, Sodium: 112mg

Ingredients:
- 4 Zucchini, small, ends trimmed
- ¼ cup Parmesan Cheese, freshly grated
- 2 Garlic cloves
- 2 tsp. Lemon Juice, fresh
- Salt & Pepper, as needed
- 2 cups Basil Leaves, fresh
- 1/3 cup Virgin Olive Oil

Instructions:
1. Slice the zucchini to noodles using a mandoline slicer or julienne peeler.
2. Place the basil and garlic in the food processor until chopped coarsely.
3. Slowly spoon in the olive oil into the food processor while it is running.
4. Open the food processor and scrape the sides using a spatula.
5. To this, spoon in the lemon juice and parmesan cheese and pulse until mixed.
6. Taste for seasoning and spoon in salt and pepper as needed.
7. Combine the zucchini and pesto in a large mixing bowl.
8. Serve and enjoy it.

Tip: If you desire, you can sauté the noodles for a few minutes in a skillet.

CAULIFLOWER FRIED RICE

Veg, Under 30 Minutes & Keto

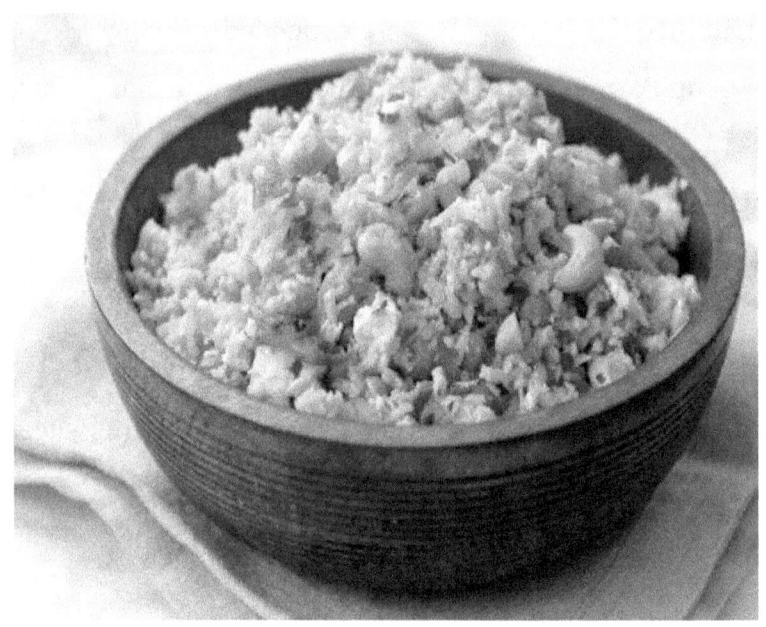

Preparation Time: 10 Minutes

Cooking Time: 15 Minutes

Efforts: Easy

Servings: 6

Nutritional Information per serving:
Calories: 135Kcal, Carbohydrates: 6.7g, Proteins: 5g, Fat: 9.3g, Sodium: 192mg

Ingredients:
- 1 Cauliflower, large
- 2 tbsp. Soy Sauce
- 2 tbsp. Butter
- Salt & Pepper, to taste
- ½ of 1 Red Pepper, chopped

- 2 Eggs, large & lightly beaten
- ½ of 1 Green Pepper, chopped
- 2 tbsp. Sesame Oil, toasted
- 2 ½ tbsp. Ginger, fresh & grated
- 3 Scallions, chopped
- 1 tbsp. Garlic, chopped

Instructions:

1. Place the cauliflower florets in a food processor and process them for 1 to 2 minutes or until riced.
2. Heat a wok over medium-high heat and spoon in butter to it.
3. Once the butter gets melted, spoon in the ginger, garlic, and pepper along with the whites of the scallions. Saute for 3 minutes.
4. Stir in the cauliflower and cook for further 3 minutes while mixing it regularly.
5. Spoon the sauce and salt over it. Mix.
6. Place the rice to one side of the pan and stir in the whisked eggs.
7. Taste for seasoning and spoon in more salt and pepper to the eggs if needed.
8. Cook for further one minute and combine it with the rest of the ingredients.
9. Spoon the sesame oil and remove from heat. Garnish with the green part of the onion.
10. Serve and enjoy it.

Tip: Pair it with roasted salmon.

CAULIFLOWER PIZZA

Veg & Keto

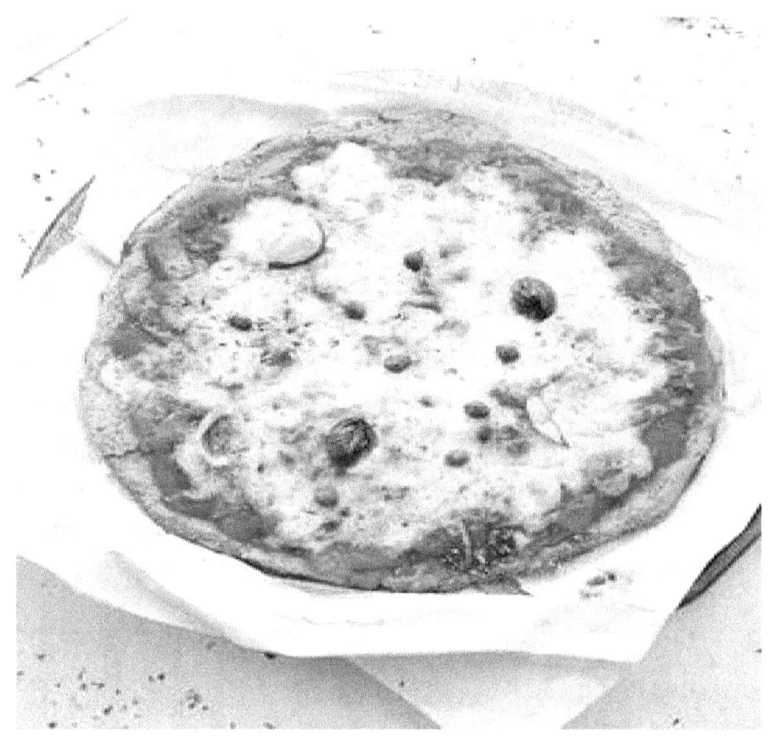

Preparation Time: 10 Minutes

Cooking Time: 20 Minutes

Efforts: Easy

Servings: 8

Nutritional Information per serving:
Calories: 99Kcal, Carbohydrates: 6g, Proteins: 8g, Fat: 6g, Sodium: 422mg

Ingredients:
- 1 Cauliflower head, medium
- ½ tsp. Basil
- ¼ cup Parmesan Cheese, shredded
- 1 Egg
- 1 cup Marinara Sauce
- ¼ cup Mozzarella Cheese
- ¼ tsp. Salt
- ½ tsp. Oregano, minced
- ½ tsp. Garlic Powder

Instructions:
1. Preheat the oven to 500° F.
2. Place the cauliflower florets in a food processor and pulse the cauliflower until it gets a riced texture.
3. Microwave the riced cauliflower in a safe microwave bowl for 5 minutes on high power.
4. Allow the riced cauliflower to cool for at least 5 to 10 minutes.
5. Once the cauliflower is cooled, place it in a cheesecloth and squeeze out all the water as much as possible.
6. Mix the cauliflower, garlic, cheese, egg, and seasoning until you get a dough-like texture.
7. Place the cauliflower dough onto a greased parchment paper-lined pizza pan.
8. Bake it for 13 to 15 minutes or until the crust is golden and crusty.
9. Top it with the marinara sauce and mozzarella cheese and return to the oven.
10. Turn on the broiler function of the oven and bake for 2 to 3 minutes or until the cheese is gooey.
11. Serve it hot. **Tip:** You can add your choice of toppings like olives, peppers, etc.

PUMPKIN SOUP

Veg & Keto

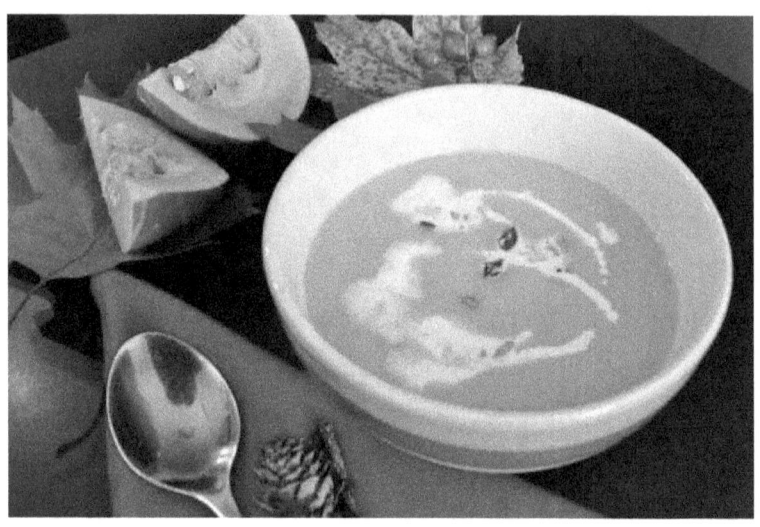

Preparation Time: 10 Minutes

Cooking Time: 30 Minutes

Efforts: Easy

Servings: 3

Nutritional Information per serving:

Calories: 610Kcal, Carbohydrates: 7.70g, Proteins: 14.44g,

Fat: 57.95g, Sodium: 657mg

Ingredients:
- 1 ½ Vegetable Broth
- 1/8 tsp. Nutmeg
- 1 cup Pumpkin Puree
- 3 tbsp. Bacon Grease
- 4 tbsp. Butter

- ½ cup Heavy Whipping Cream
- ¼ of 1 Onion, medium & chopped
- 1 Bay Leaf, large
- 2 Garlic cloves, roasted & minced
- ¼ tsp. Cinnamon
- ½ tsp. Salt & Pepper
- ¼ tsp. Coriander
- ½ tsp. Ginger, fresh & minced

Instructions:

1. Melt butter in a large saucepan over medium-low heat.
2. Once the butter is dark-golden brown colour, stir in the onions, ginger, and garlic to the pan.
3. Saute for 3 minutes and then spoon in the spices. Combine and cook for further 2 minutes.
4. Pour the vegetable broth and pumpkin puree to the pan. Mix.
5. Bring the soup to a simmer for 20 minutes after lowering the heat. Remove from heat.
6. Transfer the mixture to an immersion blender or blender once slightly cooled.
7. Blend the soup until it is completely smooth and pureed.
8. Return the soup to the pan and cook for another 20 minutes.
9. Pour the cream and bacon grease to it.
10. Serve hot.

Tip: You can top it with cooked chopped bacon if desired.

KALE SALAD

Veg, Diary-Free & Under 30 Minutes

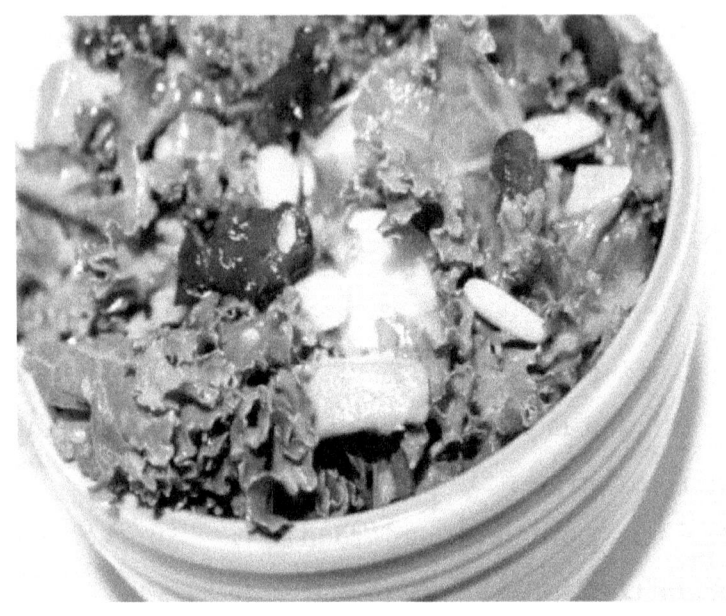

Preparation Time: 10 Minutes

Cooking Time: 5 Minutes

Efforts: Easy

Servings: 6

Nutritional Information per serving:
Calories: 242Kcal, Carbohydrates: 6g, Proteins: 6g,

Fat: 21g, Sodium: 117mg

Ingredients:
- 1/3 cup Nuts & Raisins
- 10 oz. Kale
- 1 Avocado, medium & cubed
- 2 tbsp. Lemon Juice
- ½ cup Cheese, shredded
- 2 Garlic cloves, minced
- ¼ tsp. Salt & Pepper
- ¼ cup Olive Oil

Instructions:
1. Place the kale in a large mixing bowl and set it aside.
2. Mix the olive oil, black pepper, lemon juice, salt, and garlic in another small bowl until combined well.
3. Spoon the dressing over the kale leaves and toss to coat.
4. With your hands, massage the dressing over the leaves if desired.
5. Add the cheese, nuts, and chopped avocado into it.
6. Serve and enjoy it.

Tip: If preferred, you can toast the nuts.

GARLIC MASHED CAULIFLOWER

Veg, Keto & Under 30 Minutes

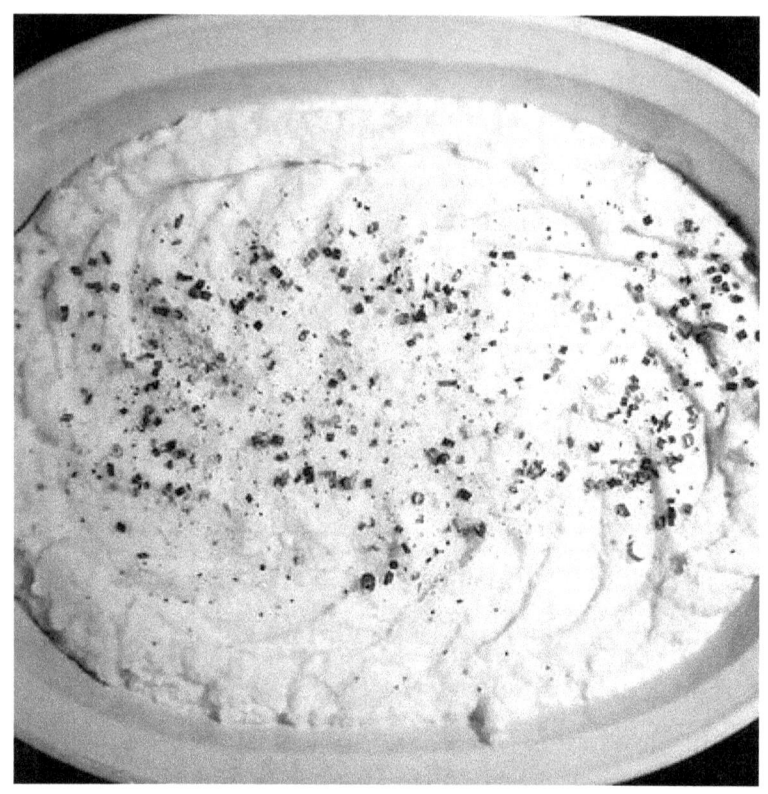

Preparation Time: 5 Minutes

Cooking Time: 5 Minutes

Efforts: Easy

Servings: 4

Nutritional Information per serving:
Calories: 126Kcal, Carbohydrates: 9g, Proteins: 6g,

Fat: 9g, Sodium: 179mg

Ingredients:

- 1 Cauliflower head, medium
- ¼ cup Parmesan Cheese
- 2 tbsp. Butter, unsalted
- 3 tbsp. Heavy Cream
- Salt & Pepper, to taste
- 3 Garlic cloves, minced

Instructions:

1. Steam the cauliflower florets in a steamer for 10 minutes or until fork-tender and soft.
2. Heat butter in a medium-soft pan over medium-high heat.
3. Once the butter has melted, stir in the garlic and saute for 1 to 2 minutes or until aromatic.
4. Take the pan off from the heat and transfer the contents to a food processor along with the cooked cauliflower, cream cheese, and parmesan.
5. Taste for seasoning and spoon in more salt and pepper if needed.
6. Blend the cauliflower mixture until it is smooth and resembles the texture of the mashed potato.
7. Serve and enjoy.

Tip: Serve it along with grilled vegetables, simple green salad for a complete meal.

GREEK SALAD

Veg, Keto & Under 30 Minutes

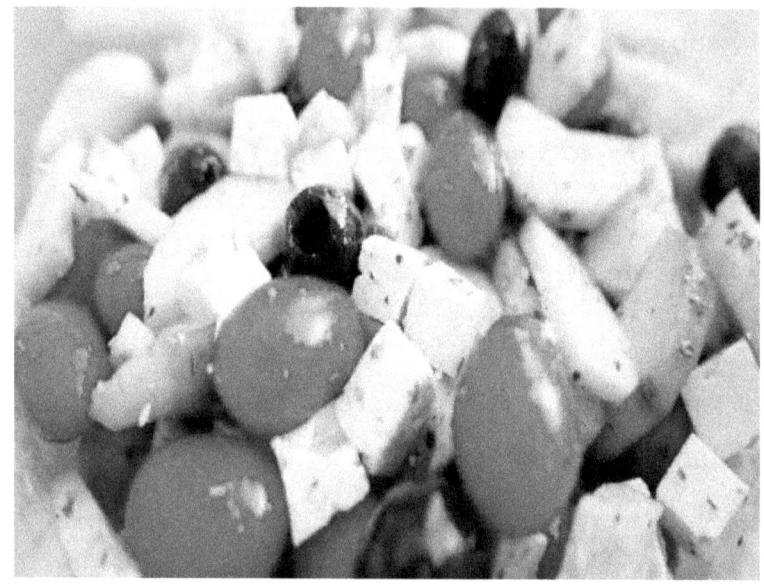

Preparation Time: 10 Minutes

Cooking Time: 10 Minutes

Efforts: Easy

Servings: 6

Nutritional Information per serving:
Calories: 117Kcal, Carbohydrates: 6g, Proteins: 4g,

Fat: 9g, Sodium: 217mg

Ingredients:

- 2 tbsp. Extra Virgin Olive Oil
- 2 Cucumbers, chopped
- 2 tbsp. Dill, fresh
- 1-pint Grape Tomatoes
- 8 to 10 Black Olives
- 4 oz. Feta Cheese

Instructions:

1. Mix all the ingredients needed to make the salad in a large mixing bowl.
2. Serve and enjoy.

Tip: Serve it along with a soup of your choice.

BROCCOLI CHEDDAR SOUP

Veg, Keto & Nut-Free

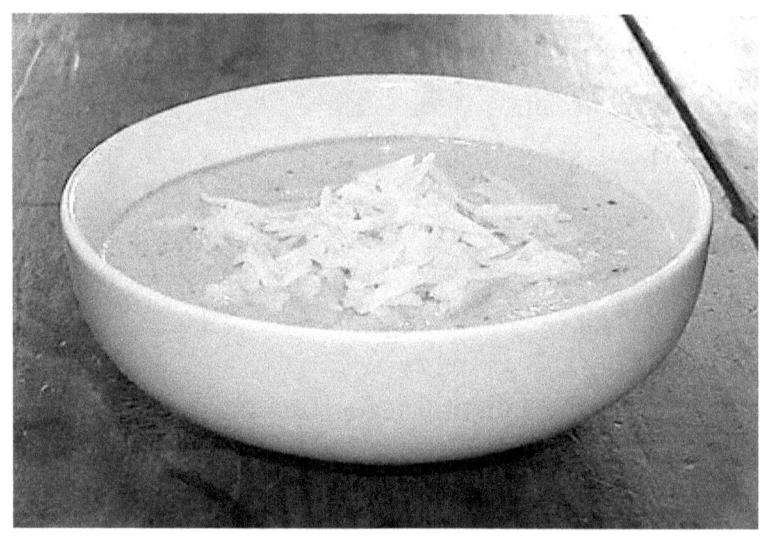

Preparation Time: 10 Minutes

Cooking Time: 20 Minutes

Efforts: Easy

Servings: 6

Nutritional Information per serving:

Calories: 255Kcal, Carbohydrates: 3g, Proteins: 7g, Fat: 22g, Sodium: 107mg

Ingredients:
- 4 cups Broccoli florets
- ¼ tsp. Black Pepper
- 2 cups Vegetable Broth
- ¼ cup Butter
- 1 cup Sharp Cheddar Cheese, shredded
- ½ cup Heavy Cream
- ½ tsp. Garlic Powder
- 1/8 tsp. Nutmeg
- ½ tsp. Onion Powder
- ½ tsp. Salt
- ½ tsp. Mustard Powder

Instructions:
1. Place the broccoli florets in a microwave-safe bowl and microwave it on 4 minutes on high power.
2. Transfer the cooked broccoli and the remaining ingredients to a high-speed blender.
3. Blend for 3 minutes or until smooth and pureed.
4. Return the soup to the bowl and microwave it again for another 2 minutes on high power.
5. Stir it well and cook for a further 2 minutes.
6. Serve hot.

Tip: You can also cook on the stovetop for 8 to 10 minutes.

ROASTED GREEN BEANS

Veg, Diary-Free & Less than 5 ingredients

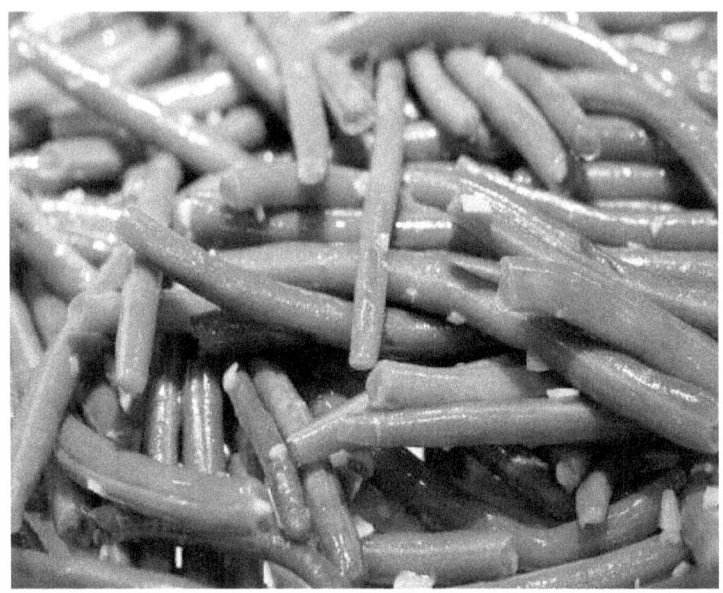

Preparation Time: 5 Minutes

Cooking Time: 25 Minutes

Efforts: Easy

Servings: 6

Nutritional Information per serving:
Calories: 73Kcal, Carbohydrates: 2g, Proteins: 7g, Fat: 5g, Sodium: 17mg

Ingredients:
- 2 tbsp. Olive Oil
- 6 cups Green Beans, raw & trimmed
- 1 tbsp. Ras El Hanout Seasoning or Moroccan Spice
- 1 tsp. Kosher Salt
- ½ tsp. Black Pepper

Instructions:
1. Mixing the green beans, seasoning, and olive oil in a mixing bowl and spread it on a greased baking sheet.
2. Roast it for 20 minutes at 400° F.
3. Once the time is up, allow it to cool for some time.
4. Return the sheet to the oven and bake for further 10 minutes.
5. Serve warm.

Tip: You can pair it with mashed cauliflower or with egg noodles.

3.3 DINNER

SALMON WITH ASPARAGUS

Keto & Under 30 Minutes

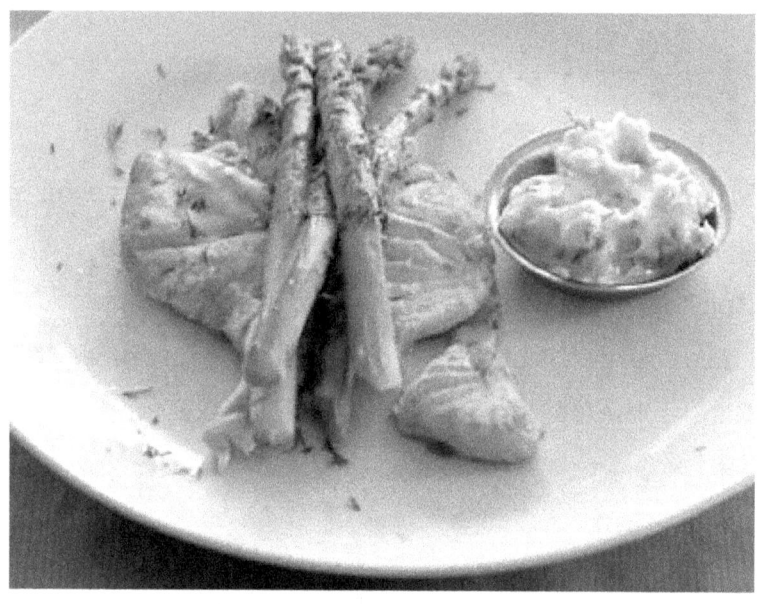

Preparation Time: 5 Minutes

Cooking Time: 10 Minutes

Efforts: Easy

Servings: 3

Nutritional Information per serving:
Calories: 409Kcal, Carbohydrates: 2.7g, Proteins: 32.8g, Fat: 28.8g, Sodium: 497mg

Ingredients:

- 1 lb. Salmon, sliced into fillets
- 1 tbsp. Olive Oil
- Salt & Pepper, as needed
- 1 bunch of Asparagus, trimmed
- 2 cloves of Garlic, minced
- Zest & Juice of ½ Lemon
- 1 tbsp. Butter, salted

Instructions:

1. Spoon in the butter and olive oil into a large pan and heat it over medium-high heat.
2. Once it becomes hot, place the salmon and season it with salt and pepper.
3. Cook for 4 minutes per side and then cook the other side.
4. Stir in the garlic and lemon zest to it.
5. Cook for further 2 minutes or until slightly browned.
6. Off the heat and squeeze the lemon juice over it.
7. Serve it hot.

Tip: You can pair it with roasted green beans also.

SHRIMP IN GARLIC BUTTER

Keto & Under 30 Minutes

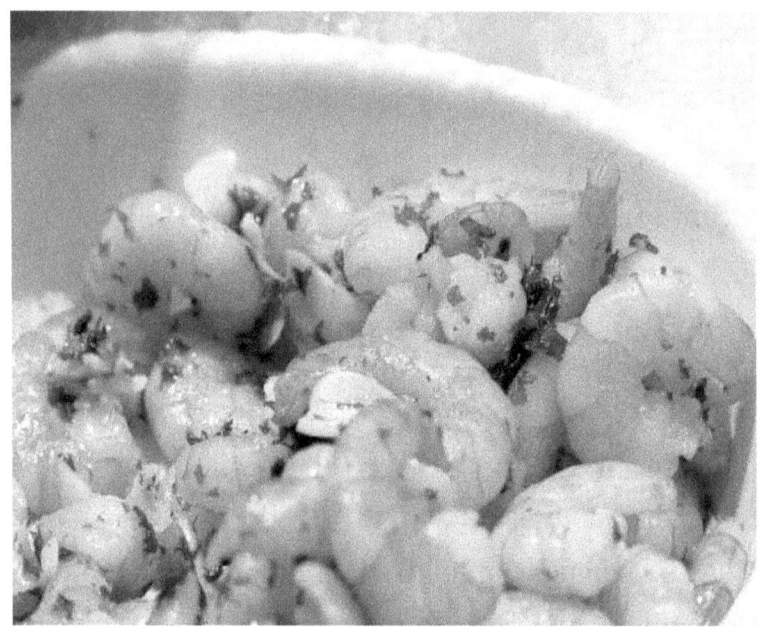

Preparation Time: 5 Minutes

Cooking Time: 20 Minutes

Efforts: Easy

Servings: 4

Nutritional Information per serving:
Calories: 307Kcal, Carbohydrates: 3g, Proteins: 27g, Fat: 20g, Sodium: 522mg

Ingredients:
- 1 lb. Shrimp, peeled & deveined
- ¼ tsp. Red Pepper Flakes
- 6 tbsp. Butter, divided
- ½ cup Chicken Stock
- Salt & Pepper, as needed
- 2 tbsp. Parsley, minced
- 5 cloves of Garlic, minced
- 2 tbsp. Lemon Juice

Instructions:
1. Heat a large bottomed skillet over medium-high heat.
2. Spoon in two tablespoons of the butter and melt it. Add the shrimp.
3. Season it with salt and pepper. Sear for 4 minutes or until shrimp gets cooked.
4. Transfer the shrimp to a plate and stir in the garlic.
5. Saute for 30 seconds or until aromatic.
6. Pour the chicken stock and whisk it well. Allow it to simmer for 5 to 10 minutes or until it has reduced to half.
7. Spoon the remaining butter, red pepper, and lemon juice to the sauce. Mix.
8. Continue cooking for another 2 minutes.
9. Take off the pan from the heat and add the cooked shrimp to it.
10. Garnish with parsley and transfer to the serving bowl.
11. Enjoy.

Tip: Serve it along with zucchini noodles.

CHICKEN CASSEROLE

Keto & Nut-free

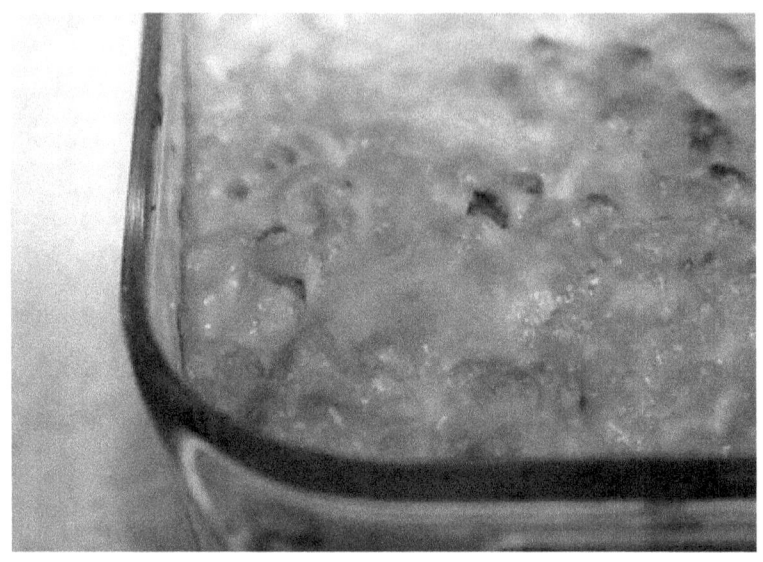

Preparation Time: 10 Minutes

Cooking Time: 45 Minutes

Efforts: Easy

Servings: 6

Nutritional Information per serving:
Calories: 672Kcal, Carbohydrates: 6g, Proteins: 36g, Fat: 56g, Sodium: 243mg

Ingredients:
- 1 cup Heavy Whipping Cream
- 4 oz. Cherry Tomatoes, sliced
- 7 oz. Cheese, shredded

- 2 tbsp. Green Pesto
- ½ of 1 Lemon, the juice
- 1 lb. Cauliflower, broken into florets.
- 30 oz. Chicken Thighs
- 3 tbsp. Butter
- 1 Leek, sliced
- Salt and Pepper, as needed

Instructions:
1. Preheat the oven to 400°F.
2. Combine cream, pesto, and lemon juice in a mixing bowl and mix well.
3. Taste for seasonings and spoon in salt and pepper.
4. Sprinkle salt and pepper over the chicken thighs.
5. Heat a large pan over medium heat and, once hot, add the butter and chicken pieces.
6. Sauté the thighs in hot butter until the meat becomes a nice golden brown.
7. Place the fried chicken thighs in a baking dish.
8. Spoon the cream mixture on top.
9. Garnish the chicken with chopped tomatoes, leek, and cauliflower.
10. Sprinkle cheese on top.
11. Bake in the oven for half an hour or until the chicken is cooked through.

Tip: You can spice it up with 1 jalapeno if desired.

COBB SALAD

Keto & Under 30 Minutes

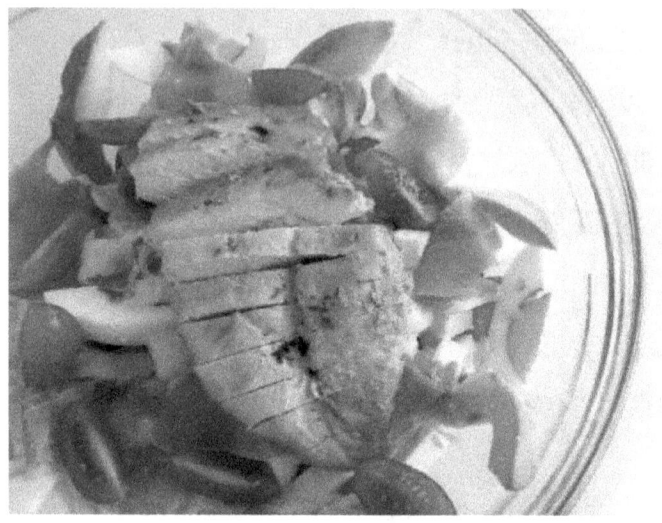

Preparation Time: 5 Minutes

Cooking Time: 5 Minutes

Efforts: Easy

Servings: 1

Nutritional Information per serving:
Calories: 307Kcal, Carbohydrates: 3g, Proteins: 27g,

Fat: 20g, Sodium: 522mg

Ingredients:
- 4 Cherry Tomatoes, chopped
- ¼ cup Bacon, cooked & crumbled
- ½ of 1 Avocado, chopped
- 2 oz. Chicken Breast, shredded
- 1 Egg, hardboiled
- 2 cups Mixed Green salad
- 1 oz. Feta Cheese, crumbled

Instructions:
1. Toss all the ingredients for the cobb salad in a large mixing bowl and toss well.
2. Serve and enjoy it.

Tip: Serve it along with mashed cauliflower or soup.

CHICKEN ENCHILADA SOUP

Keto & Nut-free

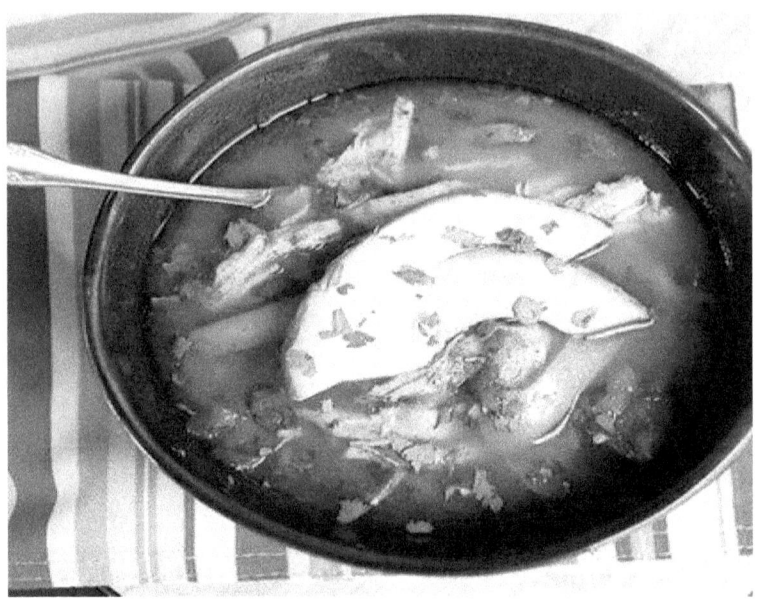

Preparation Time: 20 Minutes

Cooking Time: 45 Minutes

Effort: Beginner

Servings: 4

Nutritional Information per serving:
Calories: 358.9 Kcal, Carbohydrates: 6g, Proteins: 13.3g,

Fat: 31.3g, Sodium: 567mg

Ingredients:
- 3 tbsp. Olive Oil
- 1 cup Tomatoes, finely diced
- 6 oz. Chicken, sliced

- ½ tsp. Cayenne Pepper
- ½ cup Cilantro, chopped
- 4 cups Chicken Broth
- Juice from ½ of 1 Lime, Medium
- 8-oz. Cream Cheese
- 3 stalks Celery, finely diced
- 1 tsp. Chilli Powder
- 2 tsp. Cumin
- 2 tsp. Garlic, finely minced
- 1 tsp. Oregano, Salt and Pepper, to taste

Instructions:

1. Spoon olive oil to a heated wide saucepan over medium-high heat.
2. When the oil becomes hot, stir in celery and pepper to it.
3. Saute the celery pepper mixture for three minutes or until cooked.
4. Add tomato to it and cook for three more minutes.
5. Stir in the spice mixture and cook until fragrant.
6. Pour the chicken broth along with the cilantro to the pan and bring the mixture to a boil.
7. Reduce the heat to low. Simmer for about 20 minutes.
8. Add the chicken, drizzle it with the lemon juice and combine until everything mixes well.
9. Serve it hot along with sliced avocado on top if desired.

Tip: For a spicy kick, you can add chopped jalapeño to the soup.

SEARED TUNA STEAK

Less than 5 ingredients & Under 30 Minutes

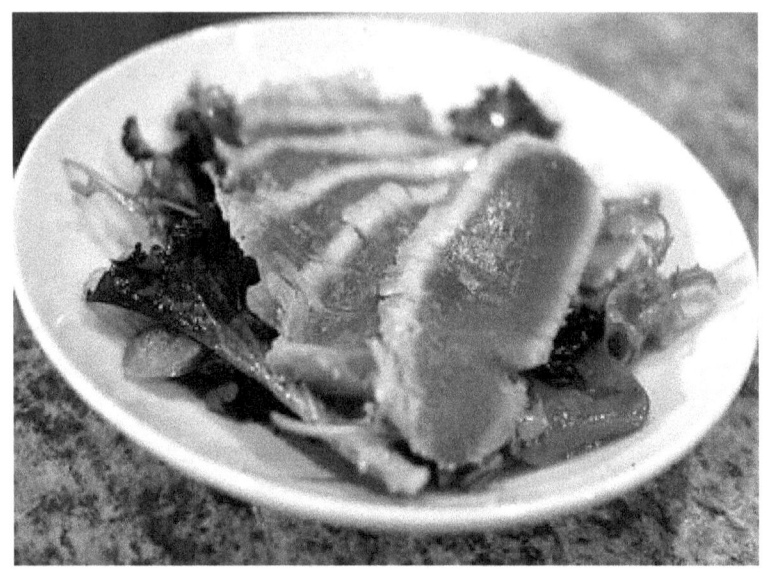

Preparation Time: 10 Minutes

Cooking Time: 10 Minutes

Effort: Easy

Serving Size: 2

Nutritional Information per serving:
Calories: 255Kcal, Carbohydrates: 1g, Proteins: 40.5g,

Fat: 9g, Sodium: 293mg

Ingredients:
- 1 tsp. Sesame Seeds
- 1 tbsp. Sesame Oil
- 2 tbsp. Soya Sauce
- Salt & Pepper, to taste
- 2 × 6 oz. Ahi Tuna Steaks

Instructions:

1. Seasoning the tuna steaks with salt and pepper. Keep it aside on a shallow bowl.
2. In another bowl, mix soya sauce and sesame oil.
3. Pour the sauce over the salmon and coat them generously with the sauce.
4. Keep it aside for 10 to 15 minutes and then heat a large skillet over medium heat.
5. Once hot, keep the tuna steaks and cook them for 3 minutes or until seared underneath.
6. Flip the fillets and cook them for a further 3 minutes.
7. Transfer the seared tuna steaks to the serving plate and slice them into ½ inch slices. Top with sesame seeds.

Tip: Pair it with a garden salad.

BRUSSELS SPROUTS WITH BACON

Under 30 Minutes & Less than 5 ingredients

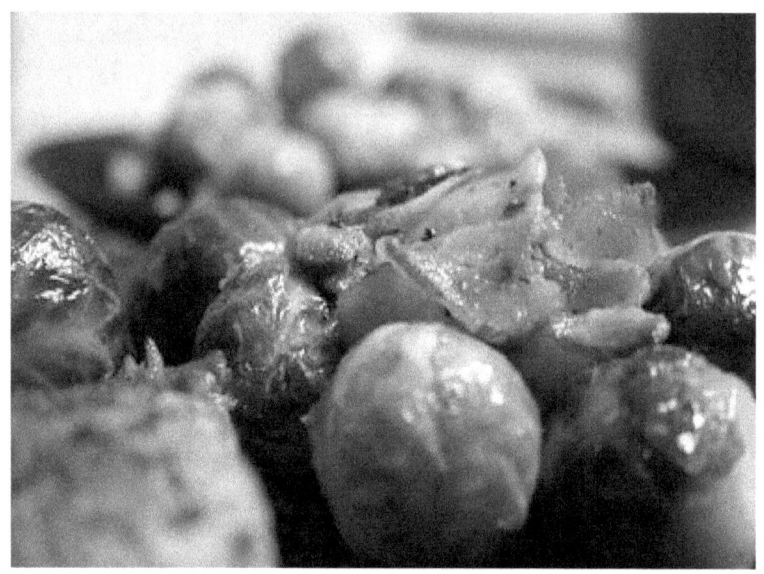

Preparation Time: 5 Minutes

Cooking Time: 25 Minutes

Effort: Easy

Serving Size: 4

Nutritional Information per serving:
Calories: 278Kcal, Carbohydrates: 4g, Proteins: 15g,

Fat: 21g, Sodium: 445mg

Ingredients:
- 8 Bacon Slices
- 1 lb. Brussels Sprouts ends trimmed & quartered
- Salt & Pepper, as needed
- 2 tbsp. Olive Oil

Instructions:
1. Preheat the oven to 375° F.
2. Combine the Brussels sprouts, olive oil, pepper, and salt in a large mixing bowl and toss them well.
3. Spread the seasoned Brussels sprouts into a greased baking sheet in a single layer.
4. Bake the sprouts for 25 to 30 minutes while turning them once in between.
5. Meantime, fry the bacon in a frying pan over medium heat.
6. When the bacon is slightly cooled, cut them into ½ inch pieces.
7. Once the Brussels sprouts are slightly blackened and shriveled, take the sheet from the oven. Mix the bacon pieces and the sprouts in a large mixing bowl and shake them well.
8. Serve and enjoy.

Tip: If desired, the Brussels sprouts can become crispier if you bake them at 400° F or 200° C.

BEEF CHILI

Keto & Diary-Free

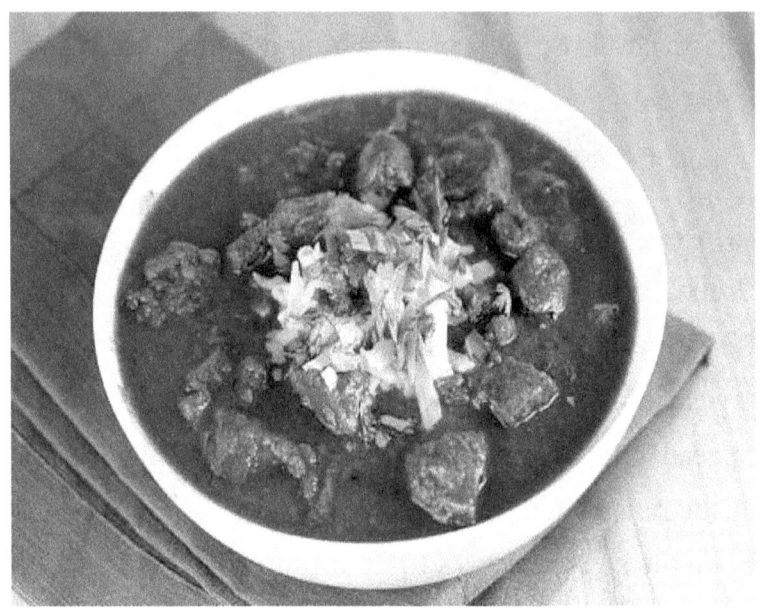

Preparation Time: 10 Minutes

Cooking Time: 20 Minutes

Effort: Easy

Serving Size: 4

Nutritional Information per serving:

Calories: 229Kcal, Carbohydrates: 2g, Proteins: 33g,

Fat: 10g, Sodium: 675mg

Ingredients:
- ½ tsp. Garlic Powder
- 1 tsp. Coriander, grounded
- 1 lb. Beef, grounded
- ½ tsp. Sea Salt
- ½ tsp. Cayenne Pepper
- 1 tsp. Cumin, grounded
- ½ tsp. Pepper, grounded
- ½ cup Salsa, low-carb & no-sugar

Instructions:
1. Heat a large-sized pan over medium-high heat and cook the beef in it until browned.
2. Stir in all the spices and cook them for 7 minutes or until everything is combined.
3. When the beef gets cooked, spoon in the salsa.
4. Bring the mixture to a simmer and cook for another 8 minutes or until everything comes together.
5. Take it from heat and transfer to a serving bowl.

Tip: You can garnish it with sour cream etc.

CHICKEN PICATTA

Keto & Nut-Free

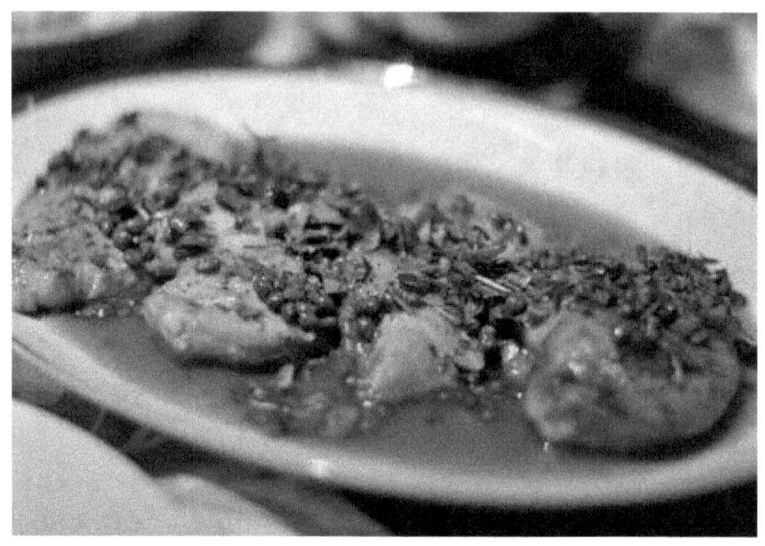

Preparation Time: 10 Minutes

Cooking Time: 15 Minutes

Effort: Easy

Serving Size: 4

Nutritional Information per serving:
Calories: 338Kcal, Carbohydrates: 4g, Proteins: 36g,

Fat: 17g, Sodium: 456mg

Ingredients:
- 2 Garlic cloves, finely minced
- ¾ cup Chicken Stock
- ¼ cup Almond Flour
- 4 × 4 Chicken Cutlets, boneless
- ¼ tsp. Black Pepper, grounded

- 4 tsp. Butter, unsalted & preferably grass-fed
- Juice from 1 Lemon
- ¼ cup Parmesan Cheese, grated
- ¼ cup Capers, drained
- 1/8 tsp. Salt
- 1 Shallot, medium & diced finely
- 4 tsp. Olive Oil

Instructions:

1. Mix parmesan cheese, pepper, almond flour, and salt on a large plate.
2. Dip the chicken cutlets in the almond flour mixture and coat the chicken thoroughly. Set it aside.
3. Heat two teaspoons of oil and butter in a large pan over medium heat.
4. Once the oil-butter starts sizzling, add the chicken pieces, and cook them for 4 minutes per side or until browned on all sides. Set it aside.
5. Spoon in the remaining oil and butter to the pan and stir in the garlic and shallot. Sauté them for a minute or two.
6. When the mixture becomes fragrant, pour in the chicken stock along with lime juice and capers. Mix well.
7. Allow it to simmer for 5 minutes or until the liquid is reduced to half.
8. Serve it hot.

Tip: For more flavour, you can substitute chicken broth with white wine.

CHICKEN NUGGETS WITH ALMOND FLOUR

Keto & Diary-Free

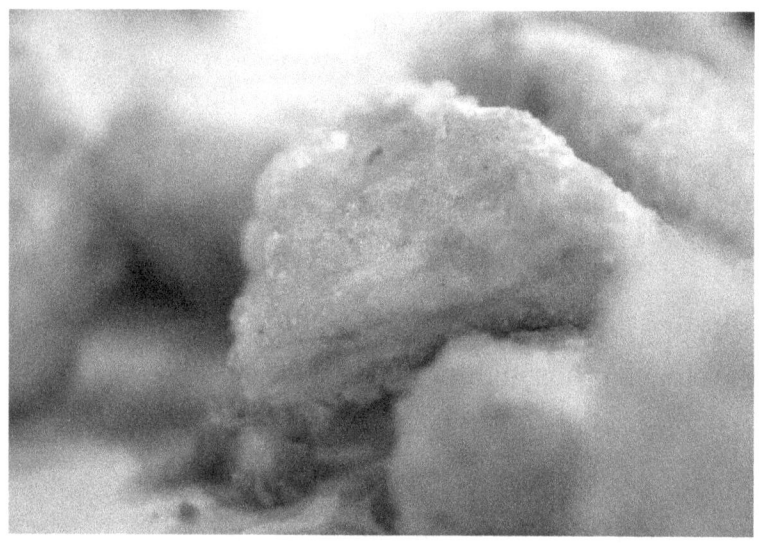

Preparation Time: 5 Minutes

Cooking Time: 25 Minutes

Efforts: Easy

Serving Size: 2

Nutritional Information per serving:
Calories: 400Kcal, Carbohydrates: 3g, Proteins: 30g, Fat: 29g, Sodium: 243mg

Ingredients:
- ½ cup Almond Meal
- Salt & Pepper, as needed
- ½ tsp. Poultry Seasoning
- 2 tbsp. Olive Oil
- 2 Chicken Breast, skinless & boneless
- 1 tsp. Paprika

Instructions:
1. Preheat the oven to 400° F.
2. Brush the oil lightly over a baking sheet and keep the baking sheet in the oven.
3. Slice each of the chicken breasts to 5 pieces. Pound them thinner if desired.
4. Combine almond meal, salt, poultry seasoning, paprika, and salt in a large mixing bowl until everything comes together.
5. Dip each of the chicken pieces to the almond meal mixture.
6. Once coated, place the chicken pieces onto the hot baking sheet and bake them for 10 minutes or until lightly browned.
7. Turn them over and bake the other side also for 10 minutes.
8. Serve it hot with mustard sauce.

Tip: If you like flaxseed meal, you can try substituting it with almond meal.

GREEK BROCCOLI SALAD

Keto & Under 30 Minutes

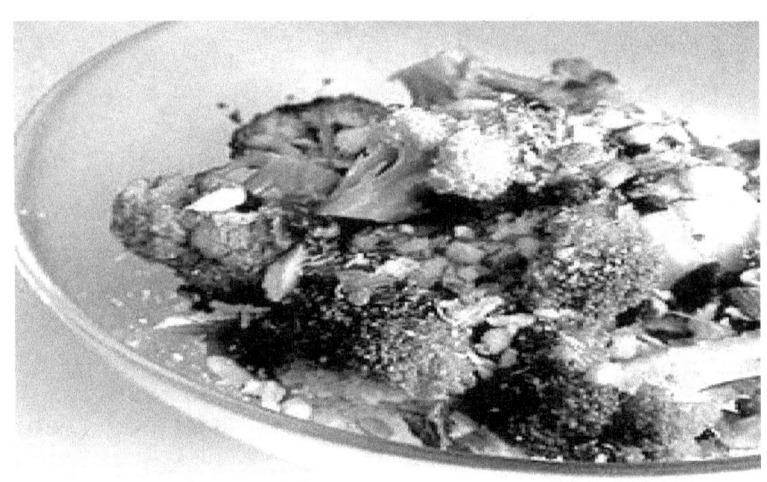

Preparation Time: 10 Minutes

Cooking Time: 15 Minutes

Efforts: Easy

Servings: 4

Nutritional Information per serving:
Calories: 272Kcal, Carbohydrates: 11.9g, Proteins: 8g,

Fat: 21.6g, Sodium: 321mg

Ingredients:
- 1 ¼ lb. Broccoli, sliced into small bites
- ¼ cup Almonds, sliced
- 1/3 cup Sun-dried Tomatoes
- ¼ cup Feta Cheese, crumbled
- ¼ cup Red Onion, sliced

For the dressing:
- 1/4 cup Olive Oil
- Dash of Red Pepper Flakes
- 1 Garlic clove, minced
- ¼ tsp. Salt
- 2 tbsp. Lemon Juice
- ½ tsp. Dijon Mustard
- 1 tsp. Low Carb Sweetener Syrup
- ½ tsp. Oregano, dried

Instructions:
1. Mix broccoli, onion, almonds and sun-dried tomatoes in a large mixing bowl.
2. In another small-sized bowl, combine all the dressing ingredients until emulsified.
3. Spoon the dressing over the broccoli salad.
4. Allow the salad to rest for half an hour before serving.

Tip: Instead of almonds, you can also use sunflower seeds.

CHEESY CAULIFLOWER GRATIN

Under 30 Minutes, Keto & Less than 5 ingredients

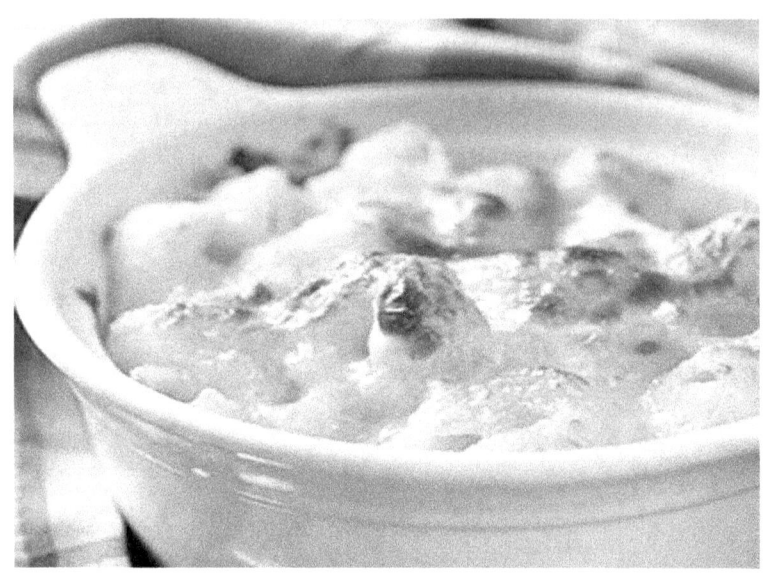

Preparation Time: 5 Minutes

Cooking Time: 25 Minutes

Efforts: Easy

Servings: 6

Nutritional Information per serving:
Calories: 421Kcal, Carbohydrates: 3g, Proteins: 19g,

Fat: 37g, Sodium: 111mg

Ingredients:

- 6 deli slices Pepper Jack Cheese
- 4 cups Cauliflower florets
- Salt and Pepper, as needed
- 4 tbsp. Butter
- 1/3 cup Heavy Whipping Cream

Instructions:

1. Mix the cauliflower, cream, butter, salt, and pepper in a safe microwave bowl and combine well.
2. Microwave the cauliflower mixture for 25 minutes on high until it becomes soft and tender.
3. Remove the ingredients from the bowl and mash with the help of a fork.
4. Taste for seasonings and spoon in salt and pepper as required.
5. Arrange the slices of pepper jack cheese on top of the cauliflower mixture and microwave for 3 minutes until the cheese starts melting.
6. Serve warm.

Tip: You can top it with nuts.

STRAWBERRY SPINACH SALAD

Keto & Less than 30 Minutes

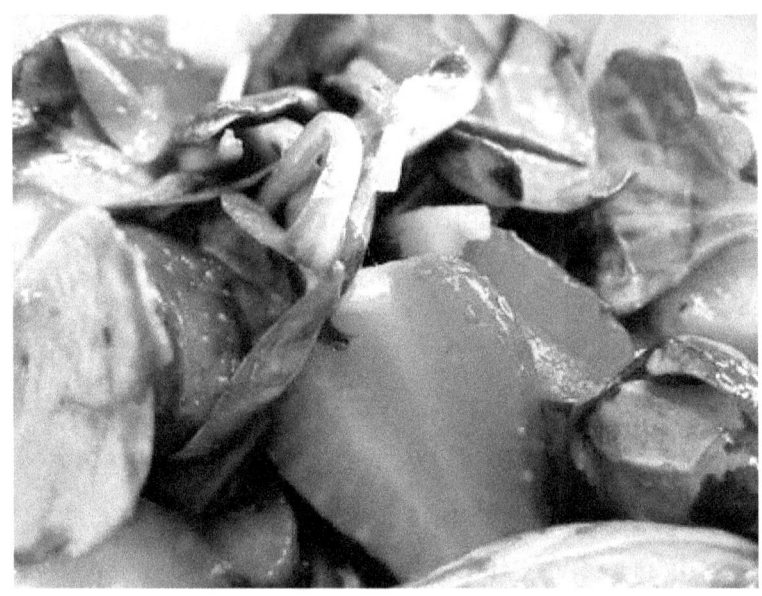

Preparation Time: 5 Minutes

Cooking Time: 10 Minutes

Efforts: Easy

Servings: 4

Nutritional Information per serving:
Calories: 255kcal, Carbohydrates: 8g, Proteins: 14g,

Fat: 16g, Sodium: 27mg

Ingredients:

- 4 oz. Feta Cheese, crumbled
- 8 Strawberries, sliced
- 2 oz. Almonds
- 6 Slices Bacon, thick-cut, crispy and crumbled
- 10 oz. Spinach leaves, fresh
- 2 Roma Tomatoes, diced
- 2 oz. Red Onion, sliced thinly

Instructions:

1. For making this healthy salad, mix all the ingredients needed to make the salad in a large-sized bowl and toss them well.

Tip: You can even add walnuts.

CAULIFLOWER MAC & CHEESE

Keto & Veg

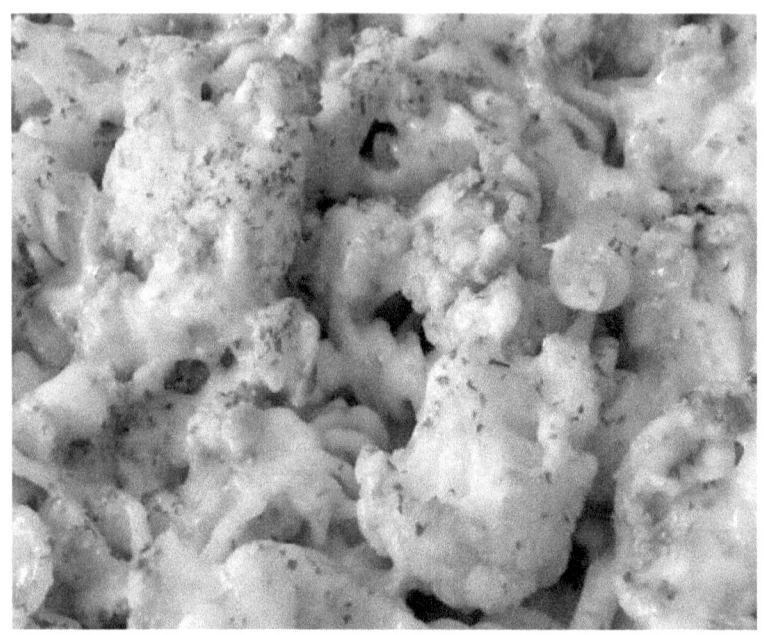

Preparation Time: 5 Minutes

Cooking Time: 25 Minutes

Effort: Easy

Serving Size: 4

Nutritional Information per serving:
Calories: 294Kcal, Carbohydrates: 7g,

Fat: 23g, Proteins: 11g

Ingredients:
- 1 Cauliflower Head, torn into florets
- Salt & Black Pepper, as needed
- ¼ cup Almond Milk, unsweetened
- ¼ cup Heavy Cream
- 3 tbsp. Butter, preferably grass-fed
- 1 cup Cheddar Cheese, shredded

Instructions:
1. Preheat the oven to 450° F.
2. Melt the butter in a small microwave-safe bowl and heat it for 30 seconds.
3. Pour the melted butter over the cauliflower florets along with salt and pepper. Toss them well.
4. Place the cauliflower florets in a parchment paper-covered large baking sheet.
5. Bake them for 15 minutes or until the cauliflower is crisp-tender.
6. Once baked, mix the heavy cream, cheddar cheese, almond milk, and the remaining butter in a large microwave-safe bowl and heat it on high heat for 2 minutes or until the cheese mixture is smooth. Repeat the procedure until the cheese has melted.
7. Finally, stir in the cauliflower to the sauce mixture and coat well.

Tip: You can add ham to it for more flavor.

EASY EGG SALAD

Veg, Under 30 Minutes & Keto

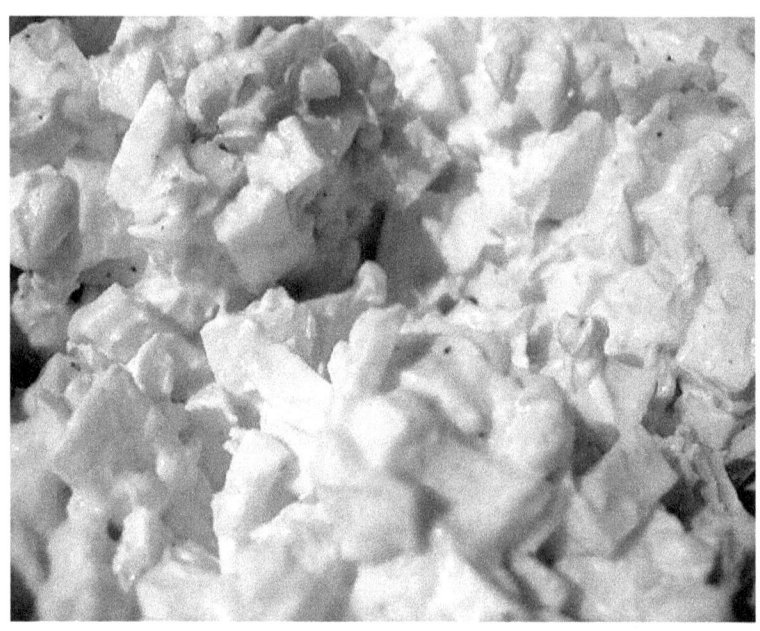

Preparation Time: 5 Minutes

Cooking Time: 15 to 20 Minutes

Effort: Easy

Servings: 4

Nutritional Information per serving:
Calories: 166kcal, Carbohydrates: 0.85g, Proteins: 10g,

Fat: 14g, Sodium: 132mg

Ingredients:
- 6 Eggs, preferably free-range
- ¼ tsp. Salt
- 2 tbsp. Mayonnaise
- 1 tsp Lemon juice
- 1 tsp Dijon mustard
- Pepper, to taste
- Lettuce leaves, to serve

Instructions:
1. Keep the eggs in a saucepan of water and pour cold water until it covers the egg by another 1 inch.
2. Bring to a boil and then remove the eggs from heat.
3. Peel the eggs under cold running water.
4. Transfer the cooked eggs into a food processor and pulse them until chopped.
5. Stir in the mayonnaise, lemon juice, salt, dijon mustard, and pepper and mix them well.
6. Taste for seasoning and add more if required.
7. Serve in the lettuce leaves.

Tip: You can place them in lettuce leaves or sandwiches.

STUFFED PEPPERS

Keto & Nut-Free

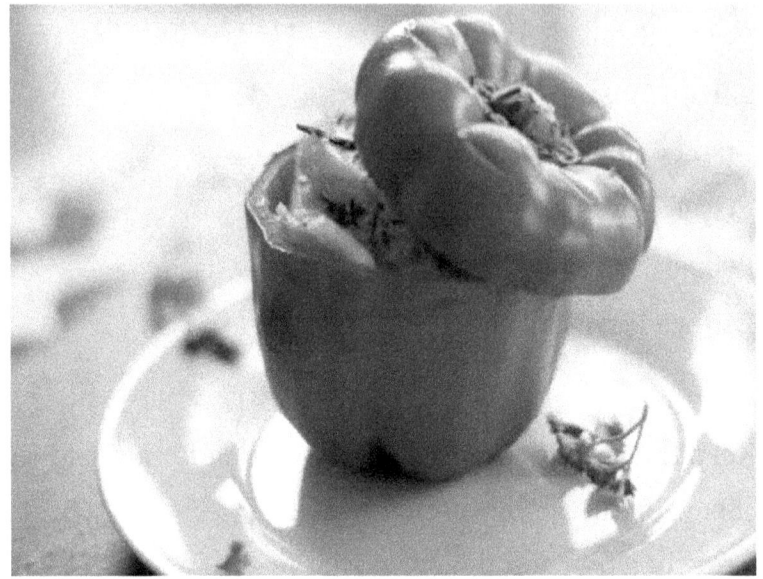

Preparation Time: 5 Minutes

Cooking Time: 25 Minutes

Effort: Easy

Servings: 6

Nutritional Information per serving:
Calories: 216kL, Carbohydrates: 4g, Protein: 16g,

Fat: 15g, Sodium: 244mg

Ingredients:
- 3 Poblano Peppers, large, tops taken off, scraped of seeds
- ¾ cup Cheddar Cheese
- 1 tbsp. Butter
- 3 oz. Cream Cheese

- 2 cloves of Garlic, minced
- 2 cups Chicken, shredded
- 2 tbsp. Taco Seasoning
- 3 oz. Cream Cheese
- 14 ½ oz. Tomatoes, diced

Instructions:
1. Preheat the oven to 350° F.
2. Place the peppers on a greased parchment paper-lined baking sheet.
3. Melt butter in a large skillet over medium heat.
4. Stir in the garlic and saute them for 30 seconds.
5. Add the chicken, taco seasoning, and diced tomatoes.
6. Bring to a boil and allow the chicken mixture to simmer for 5 minutes or until all the liquid is absorbed.
7. Lower the heat to low and spoon in the cream cheese. Stir with the back of the spatula, so everything is mixed.
8. Once combined, spoon in the chicken cheese mixture to the peppers. Top it with shredded cheese.
9. Bake for 18 minutes or until the peppers are soft, and cheese gets melted.
10. Serve it hot.

Tip: Garnish with cilantro if desired.

BAKED CHICKEN LEGS

Keto, Diary-Free & Nut-Free

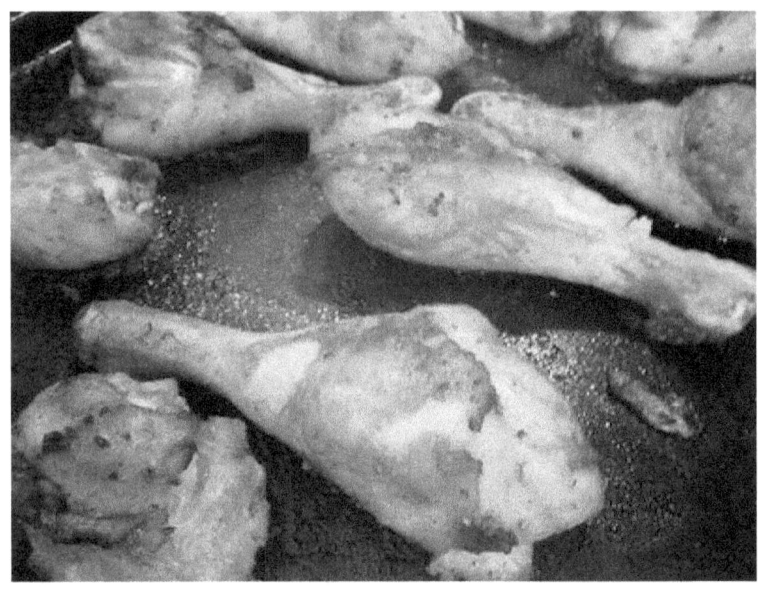

Preparation Time: 10 Minutes

Cooking Time: 40 Minutes

Effort: Easy

Servings: 6

Nutritional Information per serving:
Calories: 236kL, Carbohydrates: 0g, Protein: 22g,

Fat: 16g, Sodium: 314mg

Ingredients:
- 6 Chicken Legs
- ¼ tsp. Black Pepper
- ¼ cup Butter
- ½ tsp. Sea Salt
- ½ tsp. Smoked Paprika
- ½ tsp. Garlic Powder

Instructions:
1. Preheat the oven to 425° F.
2. Pat the chicken legs with a paper towel to absorb any excess moisture.
3. Marinate the chicken pieces by first applying the butter over them and then with the seasoning. Set it aside for a few minutes.
4. Bake them for 25 minutes. Turn over and bake for further 10 minutes or until the internal temperature reaches 165° F.
5. Serve them hot.

Tip: Serve with a spicy dipping sauce.

CREAMED SPINACH

Veg, Keto & Less than 30 Minutes

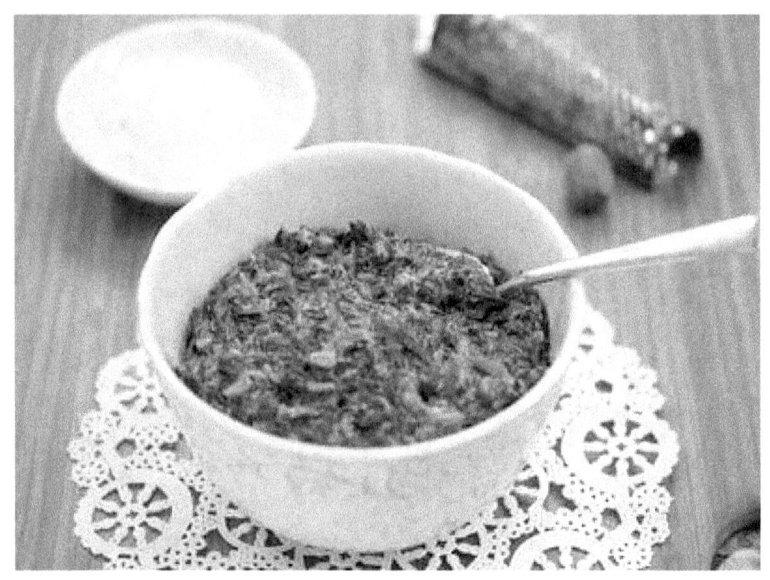

Preparation Time: 5 Minutes

Cooking Time: 10 Minutes

Effort: Easy

Servings: 4

Nutritional Information per serving:
Calories: 274kL, Carbohydrates: 4g, Protein: 4g,

Fat: 27g, Sodium: 114mg

Ingredients:
- 3 tbsp. Butter
- ¼ tsp. Black Pepper
- 4 cloves of Garlic, minced
- ¼ tsp. Sea Salt
- 10 oz. Baby Spinach, chopped
- 1 tsp. Italian Seasoning
- ½ cup Heavy Cream
- 3 oz. Cream Cheese

Instructions:
1. Melt butter in a large saute pan over medium heat.
2. Once the butter has melted, spoon in the garlic and saute for 30 seconds or until aromatic.
3. Spoon in the spinach and cook for 3 to 4 minutes or until wilted.
4. Add all the remaining ingredients to it and continuously stir until the cream cheese melts and the mixture gets thickened.
5. Serve hot

Tip: Top it with parmesan cheese if preferred.

STUFFED MUSHROOMS

Keto & Less than 5 Ingredients

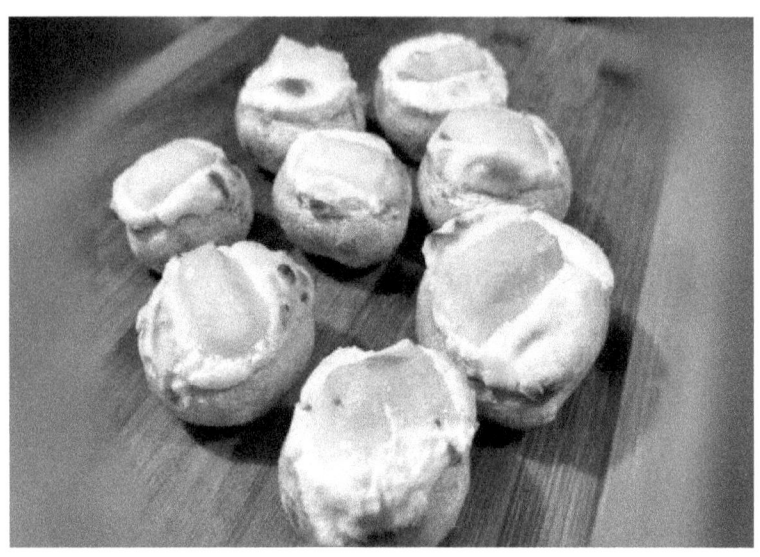

Preparation Time: 10 Minutes

Cooking Time: 20 Minutes

Effort: Easy

Servings: 4

Nutritional Information per serving:

Calories: 113kL, Carbohydrates: 4g, Protein: 7g,

Fat: 6g, Sodium: 14mg

Ingredients:
- 4 Portobello Mushrooms, large
- ½ cup Mozzarella Cheese, shredded
- ½ cup Marinara, low-sugar
- Olive Oil Spray

Instructions:
1. Preheat the oven to 375° F.
2. Take out the dark gills from the mushrooms with the help of a spoon.
3. Keep the mushroom stem upside down and spoon it with two tablespoons of marinara sauce and mozzarella cheese.
4. Bake for 18 minutes or until the cheese is bubbly.

Tip: If desired, you can pre-bake the mushrooms before filling it.

VEGETABLE SOUP

Veg, Nut-Free & Paleo

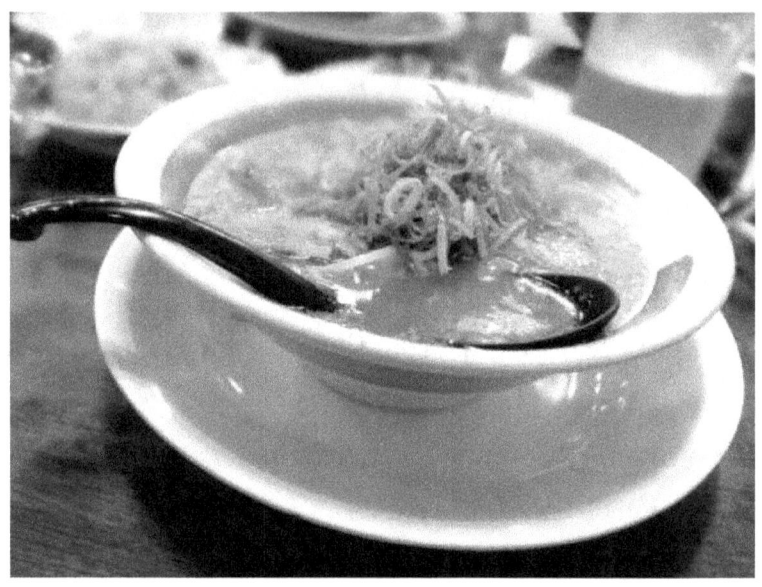

Preparation Time: 10 Minutes

Cooking Time: 30 Minutes

Effort: Easy

Servings: 5

Nutritional Information per serving:
Calories: 79kL, Carbohydrates: 8g, Protein: 2g,

Fat: 2g, Sodium: 187mg

Ingredients:
- 8 cups Vegetable Broth
- 2 tbsp. Olive Oil

- 1 tbsp. Italian Seasoning
- 1 Onion, large & diced
- 2 Bay Leaves, dried
- 2 Bell Pepper, large & diced
- Sea Salt & Black Pepper, as needed
- 4 cloves of Garlic, minced
- 28 oz. Tomatoes, diced
- 1 Cauliflower head, medium & torn into florets
- 2 cups Green Beans, trimmed & chopped

Instructions:

1. Heat oil in a Dutch oven over medium heat.
2. Once the oil becomes hot, stir in the onions and pepper.
3. Cook for 10 minutes or until the onion is softened and browned.
4. Spoon in the garlic and saute for a minute or until fragrant.
5. Add all the remaining ingredients to it. Mix until everything comes together.
6. Bring the mixture to a boil. Lower the heat and cook for further 20 minutes or until the vegetables have softened.
7. Serve hot.

Tip: If desired, you can add shredded chicken to make it more filling.

3.4 SMOOTHIES & JUICES

STRAWBERRY SMOOTHIE

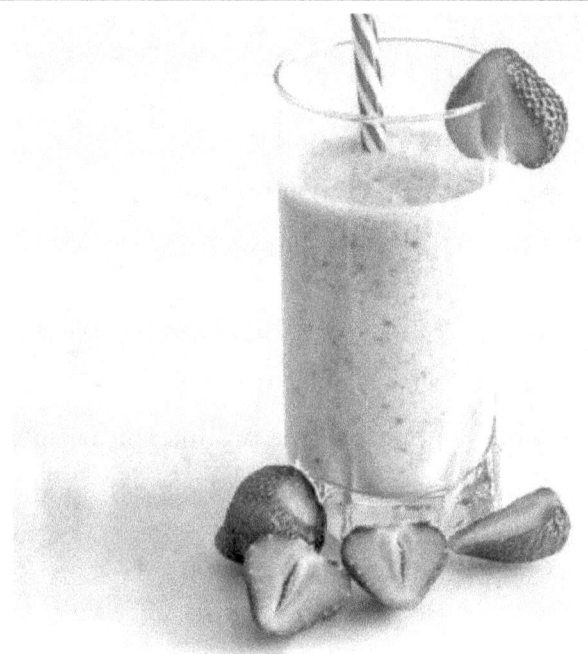

Preparation Time: 5 Minutes

Cooking Time: 5 Minutes

Efforts: Easy

Servings: 1

Nutritional Information per serving:
Calories: 167Kcal, Carbohydrates: 11g, Proteins: 16g,

Fat: 6g, Sodium: 161mg

Ingredients:
- 5 Strawberries, medium
- 6 Ice Cubes
- 1 cup Soy Milk, unsweetened
- ½ cup Greek Yoghurt, low-fat

Instructions:
1. Place strawberries, yogurt, milk, and ice cubes in a high-speed blender.
2. Blend them for 2 to 3 minutes or until you get a smooth and luscious smoothie.
3. Transfer to a serving glass and enjoy it.

Tip: You can add flax seeds or chia seeds if you prefer to make it more nutritious.

BERRY MINT SMOOTHIE

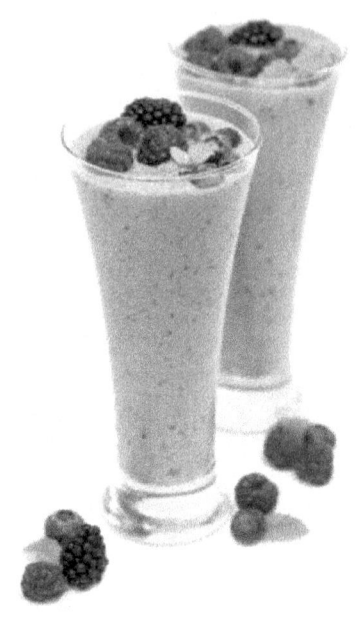

Preparation Time: 5 Minutes

Cooking Time: 5 Minutes

Efforts: Easy

Servings: 2

Nutritional Information per serving:

Calories: 137Kcal, Carbohydrates: 11g, Proteins: 6g,

Fat: 1g, Sodium: 64mg

Ingredients:

- 1 tbsp. Low-carb Sweetener of your choice
- 1 cup Kefir or Low Fat-Yoghurt
- 2 tbsp. Mint
- ¼ cup Orange
- 1 cup Mixed Berries

Instructions:

1. Place all the ingredients needed to make the smoothie in a high-speed blender and blend until smooth.
2. Transfer the smoothie to a serving glass and enjoy it.

Tip: You can add flax seeds or chia seeds if you prefer to make it more nutritious.

GREENIE SMOOTHIE

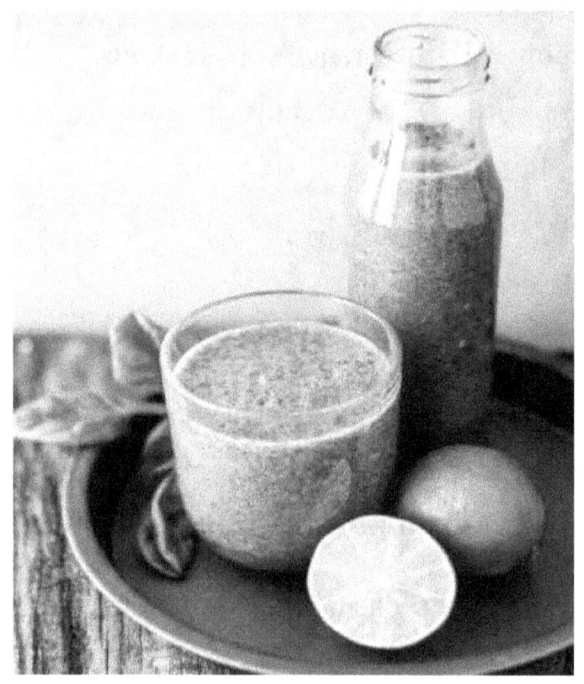

Preparation Time: 5 Minutes

Cooking Time: 5 Minutes

Efforts: Easy

Servings: 2

Nutritional Information per serving:

Calories: 123Kcal, Carbohydrates: 27g, Proteins: 2g,

Fat: 2g, Sodium: 30mg

Ingredients:
- 1 ½ cup Water
- 1 tsp. Stevia
- 1 Green Apple, ripe
- 1 tsp. Stevia
- 1 Green Pear, chopped into chunks
- 1 Lime
- 2 cups Kale, fresh
- ¾ tsp. Cinnamon
- 12 Ice Cubes
- 20 Green Grapes
- ½ cup Mint, fresh

Instructions:

1. Pour water, kale, and pear in a high-speed blender and blend them for 2 to 3 minutes until mixed.
2. Stir in all the remaining ingredients into it and blend until it becomes smooth.
3. Transfer the smoothie to serving glass.

Tip: You can stir in a teaspoon of stevia if needed.

COCONUT SPINACH SMOOTHIE

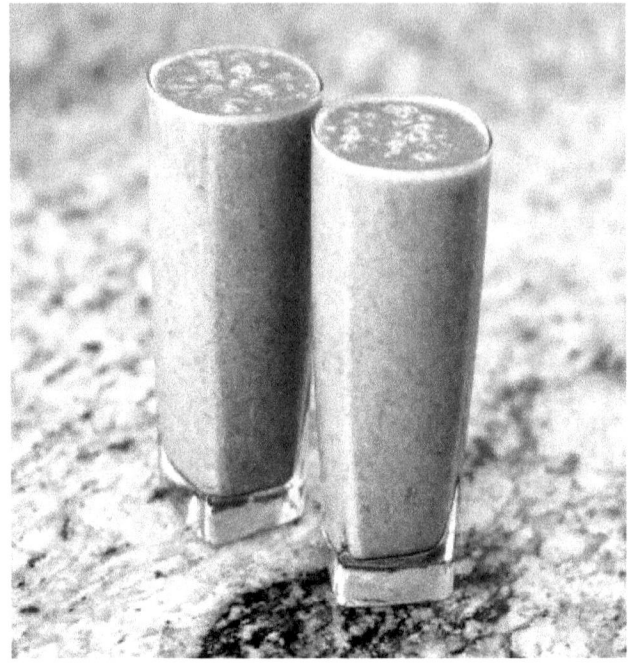

Preparation Time: 5 Minutes

Cooking Time: 5 Minutes

Efforts: Easy

Servings: 2

Nutritional Information per serving:

Calories: 251Kcal, Carbohydrates: 10.9g, Proteins: 20.3g,

Fat: 15.1g, Sodium: 102mg

Ingredients:
- 1 ¼ cup Coconut Milk
- 2 Ice Cubes
- 2 tbsp. Chia Seeds
- 1 scoop of Protein Powder, preferably vanilla
- 1 cup Spin

Instructions:

1. Pour coconut milk along with spinach, chia seeds, protein powder, and ice cubes in a high-speed blender.
2. Blend for 2 minutes to get a smooth and luscious smoothie.
3. Serve in a glass and enjoy it.

Tip: You can avoid protein powder if not desired.

OATS COFFEE SMOOTHIE

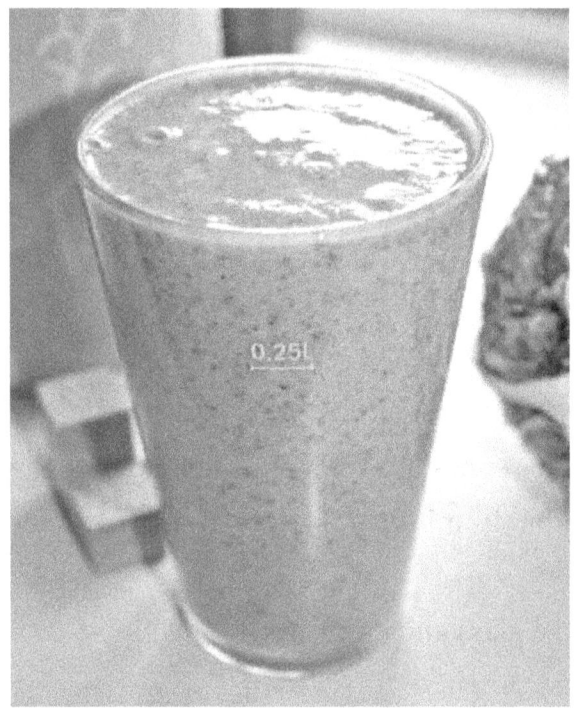

Preparation Time: 5 Minutes

Cooking Time: 5 Minutes

Efforts: Easy

Servings: 2

Nutritional Information per serving:
Calories: 251Kcal, Carbohydrates: 10.9g, Proteins: 20.3g,

Fat: 15.1g, Sodium: 102mg

Ingredients:

- 1 cup Oats, uncooked & grounded
- 2 tbsp. Instant Coffee
- 3 cup Milk, skimmed
- 2 Banana, frozen & sliced into chunks
- 2 tbsp. Flax Seeds, grounded

Instructions:

1. Place all the ingredients in a high-speed blender and blend for 2 minutes or until smooth and luscious.
2. Serve and enjoy.

Tip: If you need more sweetness, one teaspoon of any low-carb sweetener.

VEGGIE SMOOTHIE

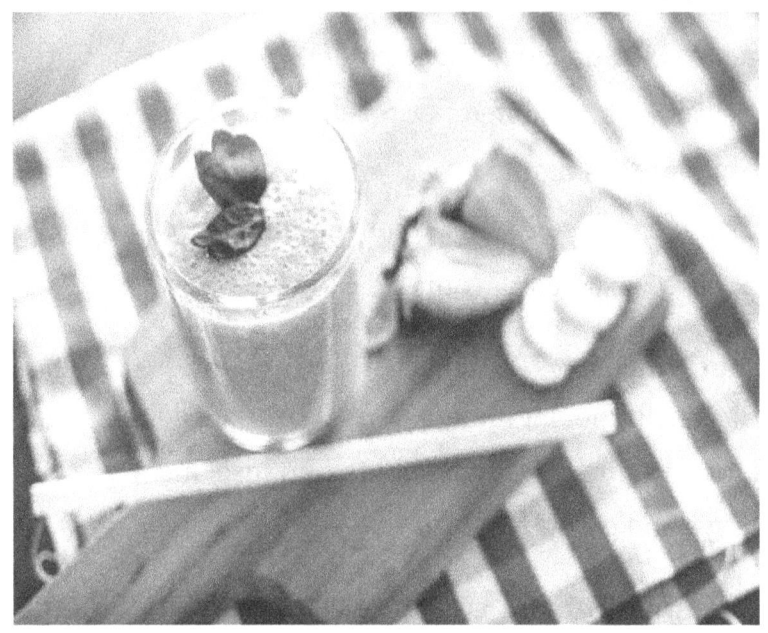

Preparation Time: 5 Minutes

Cooking Time: 5 Minutes

Efforts: Easy

Servings: 1

Nutritional Information per serving:
Calories: 169cal, Carbohydrates: 17g, Proteins: 2.3g,

Fat: 9.8g, Sodium: 162mg

Ingredients:
- ¼ of 1 Red Bell Pepper, sliced
- ½ tbsp. Coconut Oil
- 1 cup Almond Milk, unsweetened
- ¼ tsp. Turmeric
- 4 Strawberries, chopped
- Pinch of Cinnamon
- ½ of 1 Banana, preferably frozen

Instructions:
1. Combine all the ingredients required to make the smoothie in a high-speed blender.
2. Blend for 3 minutes to get a smooth and silky mixture.
3. Serve and enjoy.

Tip: If you need more sweetness, one teaspoon of any low-carb sweetener.

AVOCADO SMOOTHIE

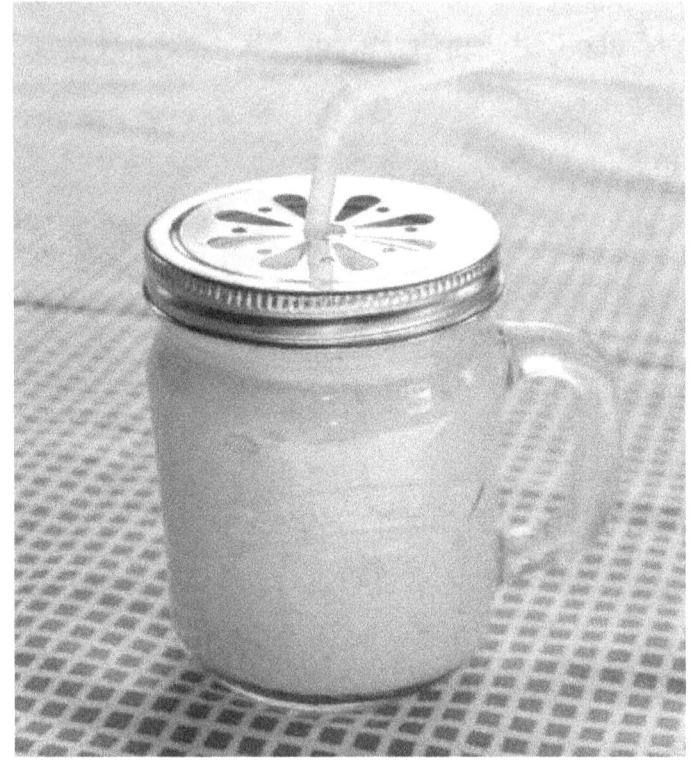

Preparation Time: 10 Minutes

Cooking Time: 0 Minutes

Efforts: Easy

Servings: 2

Nutritional Information per serving:
Calories: 214cal, Carbohydrates: 15g, Proteins: 2g,

Fat: 17g, Sodium: 25mg

Ingredients:

- 1 Avocado, ripe & pit removed
- 2 cups Baby Spinach
- 2 cups Water
- 1 cup Baby Kale
- 1 tbsp. Lemon Juice
- 2 sprigs of Mint
- ½ cup Ice Cubes

Instructions:

1. Place all the ingredients needed to make the smoothie in a high-speed blender and blend until smooth.
2. Transfer to a serving glass and enjoy it.

Tip: If you want to add more sweetness, you can add a pinch of honey.

ORANGE CARROT SMOOTHIE

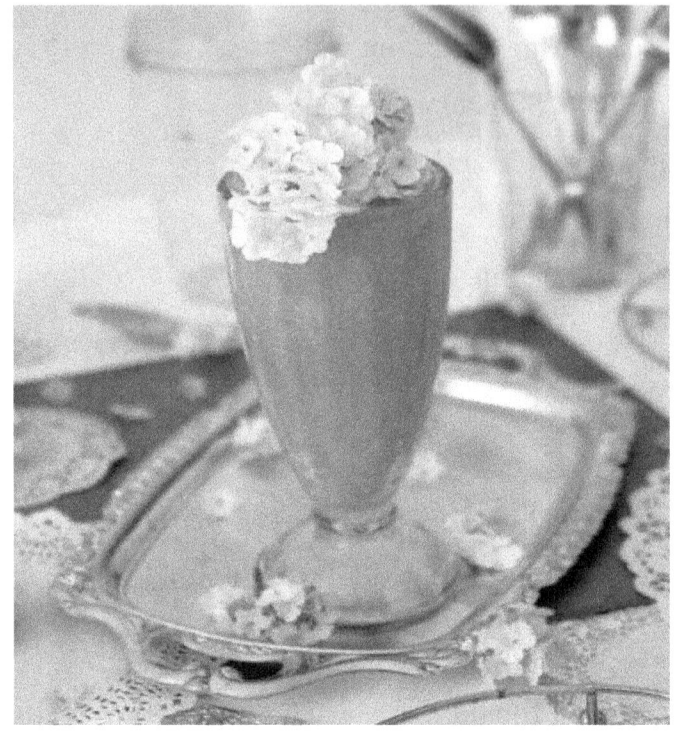

Preparation Time: 5 Minutes

Cooking Time: 0 Minutes

Efforts: Easy

Servings: 1

Nutritional Information per serving:
Calories: 216cal, Carbohydrates: 10g, Proteins: 15g,

Fat: 7g, Sodium: 25mg

Ingredients:

- 1 ½ cups Almond Milk
- ¼ cup Cauliflower, blanched & frozen
- 1 Orange
- 1 tbsp. Flax Seed
- 1/3 cup Carrot, grated
- 1 tsp. Vanilla Extract

Instructions:

1. Mix all the ingredients in a high-speed blender and blend for 2 minutes or until you get the desired consistency.
2. Transfer to a serving glass and enjoy it.

Tip: If you want to make it more nutritious, you can add collagen powder.

BLACKBERRY SMOOTHIE

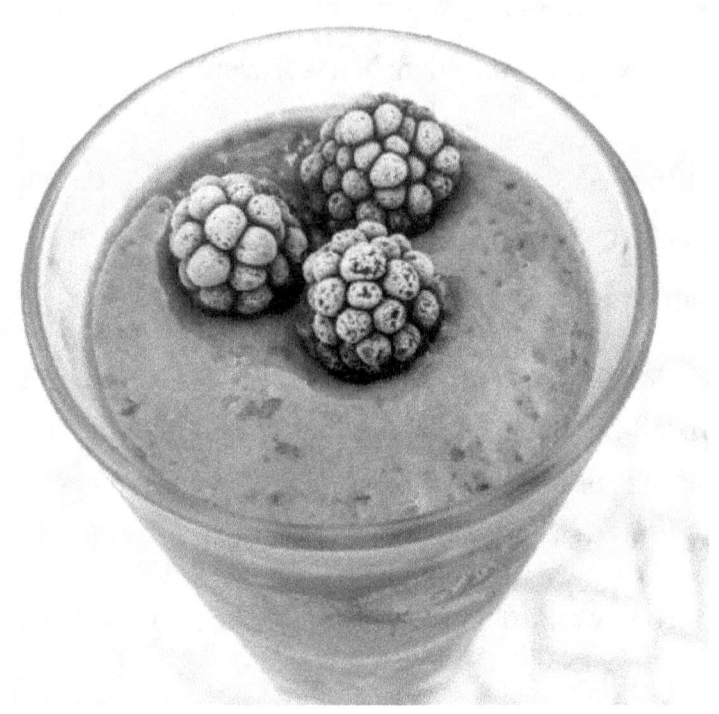

Preparation Time: 5 Minutes

Cooking Time: 0 Minutes

Efforts: Easy

Servings: 1

Nutritional Information per serving:
Calories: 275cal, Carbohydrates: 9g, Proteins: 11g,

Fat: 17g, Sodium: 73mg

Ingredients:

- 1 ½ cups Almond Milk
- ¼ cup Cauliflower, blanched & frozen
- 1 Orange
- 1 tbsp. Flax Seed
- 1/3 cup Carrot, grated
- 1 tsp. Vanilla Extract

Instructions:

1. Place all the ingredients needed to make the blackberry smoothie in a high-speed blender and blend for 2 minutes until you get a smooth mixture.
2. Transfer to a serving glass and enjoy it.

Tip: Instead of cauliflower, you can also use blanched & frozen zucchini.

KEY LIME PIE SMOOTHIE

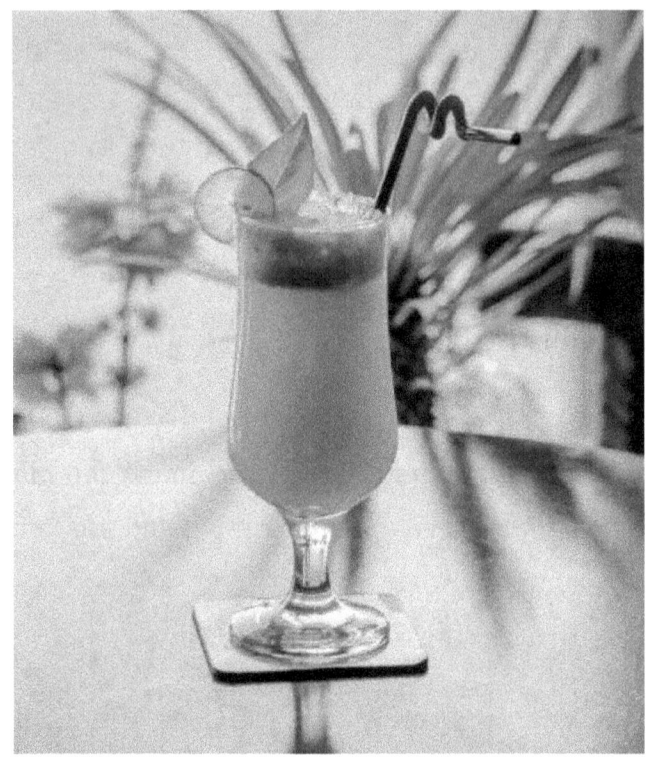

Preparation Time: 5 Minutes

Cooking Time: 0 Minutes

Efforts: Easy

Servings: 1

Nutritional Information per serving:
Calories: 180cal, Carbohydrates: 7g, Proteins: 36g,

Fat: 1g, Sodium: 35mg

Ingredients:
- ½ cup Cottage Cheese
- 1 tbsp. Sweetener of your choice
- ½ cup Water
- ½ cup Spinach
- 1 tbsp. Lime Juice
- 1 cup Ice Cubes

Instructions:

1. Spoon in the ingredients to a high-speed blender and blend until silky smooth.
2. Transfer to a serving glass and enjoy it.

Tip: Instead of water, you can use almond milk to make it more nutritious and creamy.

CINNAMON ROLL SMOOTHIE

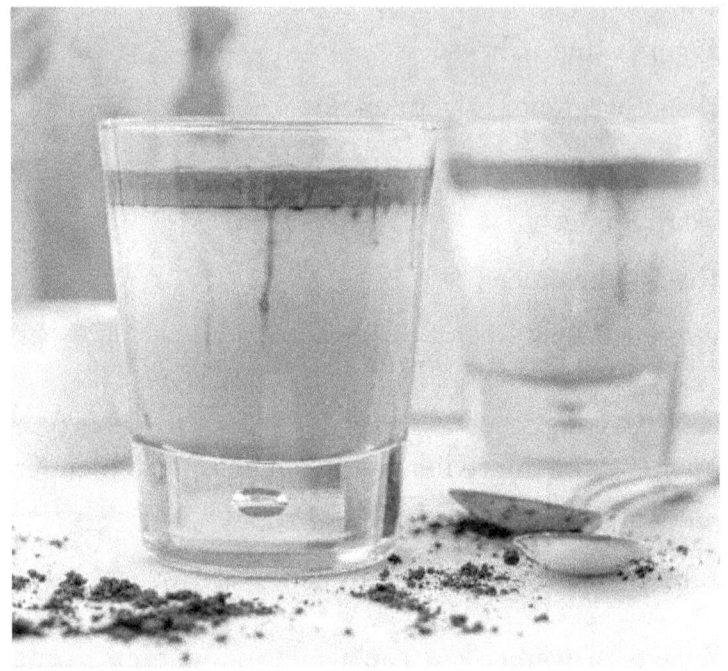

Preparation Time: 5 Minutes

Cooking Time: 0 Minutes

Efforts: Easy

Servings: 1

Nutritional Information per serving:
Calories: 145cal, Carbohydrates: 1.6g, Proteins: 26.5g, Fat: 3.25g, Sodium: 30mg

Ingredients:
- 1 tsp. Flax Meal or oats, if preferred
- 1 cup Almond Milk
- ½ tsp. Cinnamon
- 2 tbsp. Protein Powder
- 1 cup Ice
- ¼ tsp. Vanilla Extract
- 4 tsp. Sweetener of your choice

Instructions:
1. Pour the milk into the blender, followed by the protein powder, sweetener, flax meal, cinnamon, vanilla extract, and ice.
2. Blend for 40 seconds or until smooth.
3. Serve and enjoy.

Tip: Instead of water, you can use almond milk to make it more nutritious and creamy.

STRAWBERRY CHEESECAKE SMOOTHIE

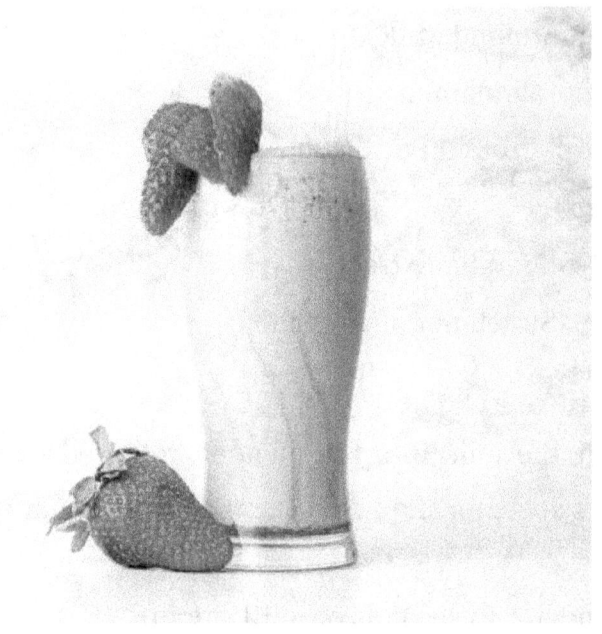

Preparation Time: 5 Minutes

Cooking Time: 0 Minutes

Efforts: Easy

Servings: 1

Nutritional Information per serving:

Calories: 347cal, Carbohydrates: 10.05g, Proteins: 17.5g, Fat: 24g, Sodium: 45mg

Ingredients:
- ¼ cup Soy Milk, unsweetened
- ½ cup Cottage Cheese, low-fat
- ½ tsp. Vanilla Extract
- 2 oz. Cream Cheese
- 1 cup Ice Cubes
- ½ cup Strawberries
- 4 tbsp. Low-carb Sweetener of your choice

Instructions:
1. Add all the ingredients for making the strawberry cheesecake smoothie to a high-speed blender until you get the desired smooth consistency.
2. Serve and enjoy.

Tip: Instead of soy milk, you can also use almond milk or water.

PEANUT BUTTER BANANA SMOOTHIE

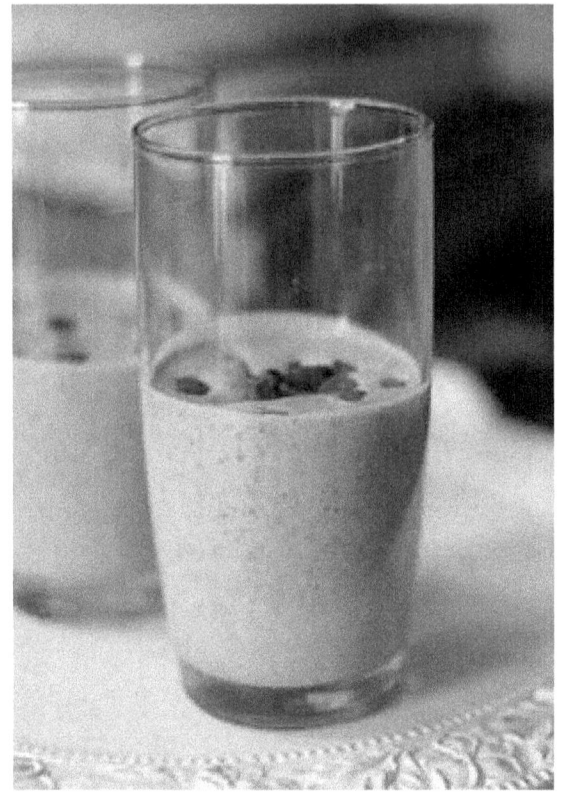

Preparation Time: 5 Minutes

Cooking Time: 2 Minutes

Efforts: Easy

Servings: 1

Nutritional Information per serving:
Calories: 202cal, Carbohydrates: 14g, Proteins: 10g, Fat: 9g, Sodium: 30mg

Ingredients:

- ¼ cup Greek Yoghurt, plain
- ½ tbsp. Chia Seeds
- ½ cup Ice Cubes
- ½ of 1 Banana
- ½ cup Water
- 1 tbsp. Peanut Butter

Instructions:

1. Place all the ingredients needed to make the smoothie in a high-speed blender and blend to get a smooth and luscious mixture.
2. Transfer the smoothie to a serving glass and enjoy it.

Tip: If desired, you can add chocolate chips to it.

AVOCADO TURMERIC SMOOTHIE

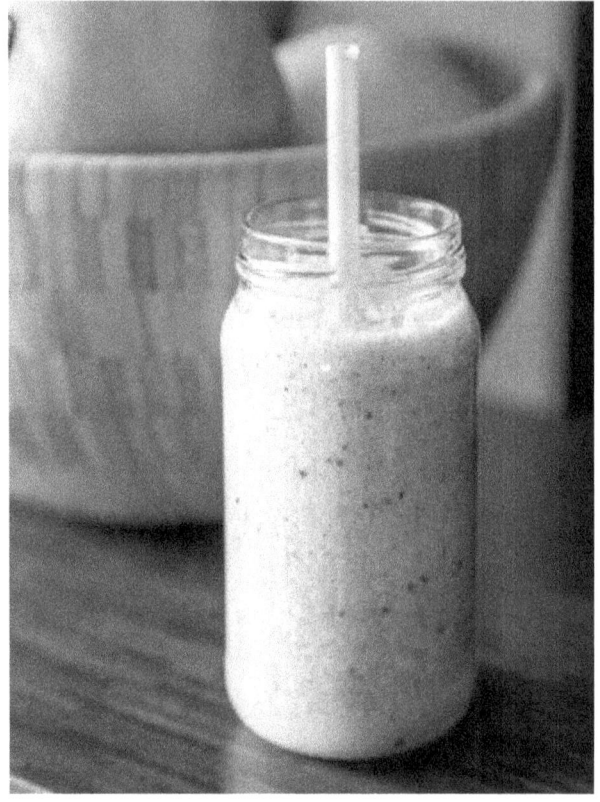

Preparation Time: 5 Minutes

Cooking Time: 2 Minutes

Efforts: Easy

Servings: 1

Nutritional Information per serving:
Calories: 232cal, Carbohydrates: 4.1g, Proteins: 1.7g,

Fat: 22.4g, Sodium: 25mg

Ingredients:

- ½ of 1 Avocado
- 1 cup Ice, crushed
- ¾ cup Coconut Milk, full-fat
- 1 tsp. Lemon Juice
- ¼ cup Almond Milk
- ½ tsp. Turmeric
- 1 tsp. Ginger, freshly grated

Instructions:

1. Place all the ingredients excluding the crushed ice in a high-speed blender and blend for 2 to 3 minutes or until smooth.
2. Transfer to a serving glass and enjoy it.

Tip: If desired, you can add a pinch of pepper to it.

BLUEBERRY SMOOTHIE

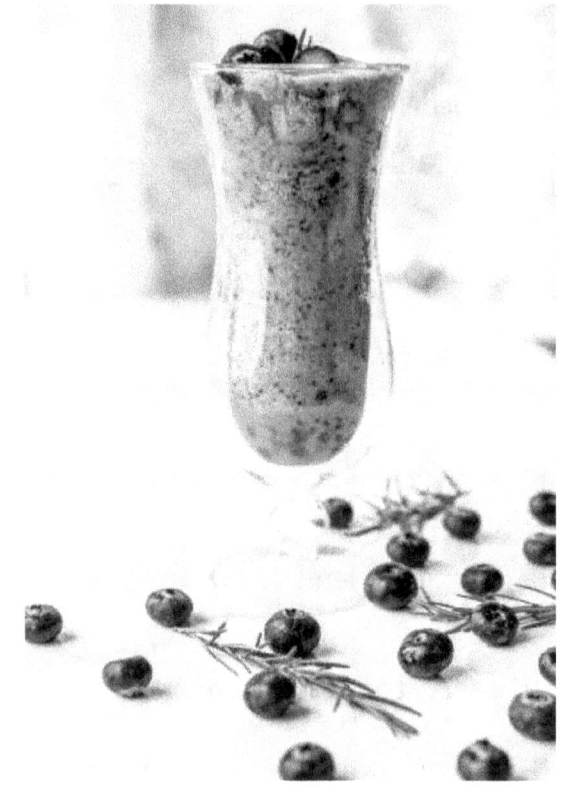

Preparation Time: 5 Minutes

Cooking Time: 2 Minutes

Efforts: Easy

Servings: 2

Nutritional Information per serving:

Calories: 417cal, Carbohydrates: 9g, Proteins: 4g,

Fat: 43g, Sodium: 35mg

Ingredients:

- 1 tbsp. Lemon Juice
- 1 ¾ cup Coconut Milk, full-fat
- ½ tsp. Vanilla Extract
- 3 oz. Blueberries, frozen

Instructions:

1. Combine coconut milk, blueberries, lemon juice, and vanilla extract in a high-speed blender.
2. Blend for 2 minutes for a smooth and luscious smoothie.
3. Serve and enjoy.

Tip: If desired, you can add more lemon juice to it for more tanginess.

MATCHA GREEN SMOOTHIE

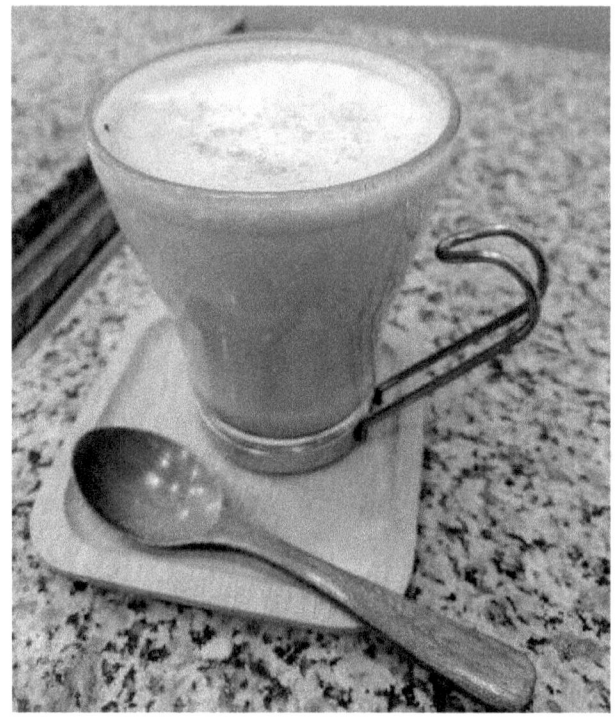

Preparation Time: 5 Minutes

Cooking Time: 2 Minutes

Efforts: Easy

Servings: 2

Nutritional Information per serving:
Calories: 229cal, Carbohydrates: 1.5g, Proteins: 14.1g,

Fat: 43g, Sodium: 35mg

Ingredients:
- ¼ cup Heavy Whipping Cream
- ½ tsp. Vanilla Extract
- 1 tsp. Matcha Green Tea Powder
- 2 tbsp. Protein Powder
- 1 tbsp. Hot Water
- 1 ¼ cup Almond Milk, unsweetened
- ½ of 1 Avocado, medium

Instructions:
1. Place all the ingredients in the high-blender for one to two minutes.
2. Serve and enjoy.

Tip: If desired, you can spoon in one to two tablespoon of swerve sweetener for sweetness.

TROPICAL SMOOTHIE

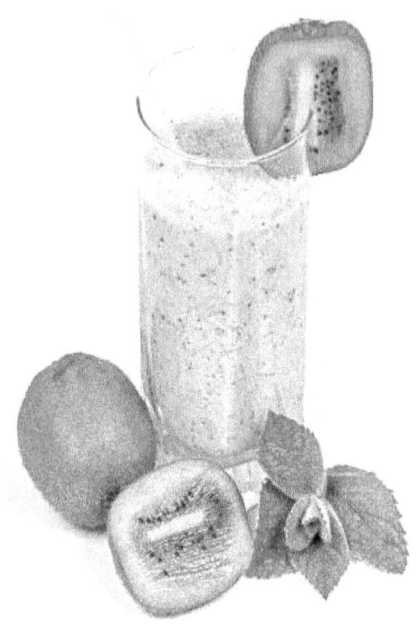

Preparation Time: 5 Minutes

Cooking Time: 2 Minutes

Efforts: Easy

Servings: 6

Nutritional Information per serving:
Calories: 37cal, Carbohydrates: 3g, Proteins: 1g,

Fat: 2g, Sodium: 10mg

Ingredients:

- 2 tbsp. Parsley, fresh
- 4 cups Water
- 1 tbsp. Granulated Low-Carb Sweetener
- 1 cup Romaine Lettuce
- ½ of 1 Avocado
- 1/3 cup Pineapple, fresh & chopped
- ½ cup Kiwi Fruit
- 1 tbsp. Ginger, fresh, peeled & chopped
- 1 cup Cucumber, peeled & sliced

Instructions:

1. Spoon in all the ingredients needed to make the smoothie in a high-speed blender for 1 to 2 minutes.
2. Blend until pureed.
3. Serve and enjoy.

Tip: If desired, you can spoon in one to two tablespoon of swerve sweetener for sweetness.

ORANGE CARROT JUICE

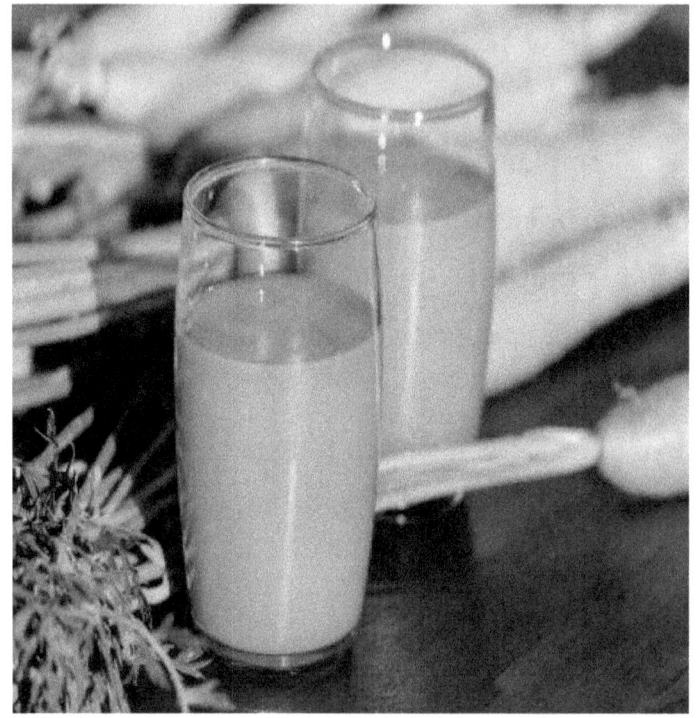

Preparation Time: 1 Minute

Cooking Time: 2 Minutes

Efforts: Easy

Servings: 1

Nutritional Information per serving:
Calories: 159cal, Carbohydrates: 27g, Proteins: 4g,

Fat: 2g, Sodium: 86mg

Ingredients:

- 1/2-inch Ginger knob
- ½ cup Almond Milk, unsweetened
- 1 Orange, large & peeled
- ½ of 1 Yellow Pepper
- 2 Carrots, large & peeled

Instructions:

1. Place all the ingredients needed to make the juice in a blender or juicer.
2. Blend for 2 minutes to get a smooth juice.
3. Serve along with ice.

Tip: If desired, you can add chocolate chips to it.

GREEN DETOX JUICE

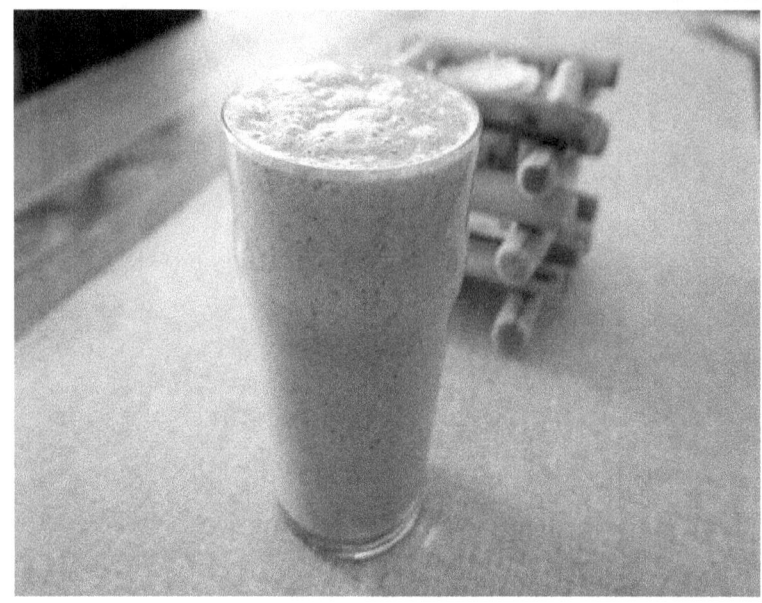

Preparation Time: 10 Minutes

Cooking Time: 2 Minutes

Efforts: Easy

Servings: 1 to 2

Nutritional Information per serving:

Calories: 157cal, Carbohydrates: 18g, Proteins: 12.3g,

Fat: 3.6g, Sodium: 304mg

Ingredients:

- 1 Lime
- 2 Cucumbers
- 1 handful of Parsley
- 1 bunch of White Celery
- 2 handful of Spinach
- 1 tsp. MCT Oil
- 1 knob of Ginger, fresh

Instructions:

1. Place all the ingredients needed to make the detox juice in a high-speed blender.
2. Blend for 2 minutes or until pureed.
3. Transfer to a serving glass and enjoy it.

Tip: If preferred, you can add 1 to 2 teaspoon more of MCT oil to make it more nutritious.

RASPBERRY LEMONADE

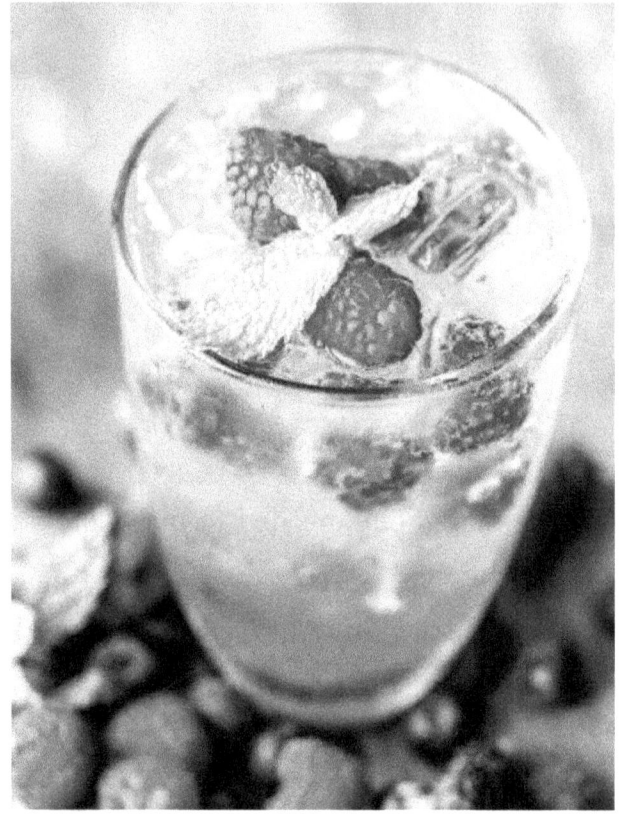

Preparation Time: 10 Minutes

Cooking Time: 2 Minutes

Efforts: Easy

Servings: 1 to 2

Nutritional Information per serving:

Calories: 107cal, Carbohydrates: 20g, Proteins: 1.7g,

Fat: 0.6g, Sodium: 10mg

Ingredients:
- 1 cup Raspberries, frozen
- 1 handful of Mint Leaves
- 2 cups Water
- 2 tbsp. Date Paste
- 2 drops of Liquid Stevia
- ¼ cup Orange Juice

Instructions:
1. Place all the ingredients in a high-speed blender or juicer.
2. Blend for 2 minutes or until pureed and smooth.
3. Serve and enjoy.

Tip: If desired, you can add raspberry extract to it.

3.5 DESSERTS

PEANUT BUTTER COOKIES

Under 30 Minutes, Diary-Free & Less than 5-ingredients

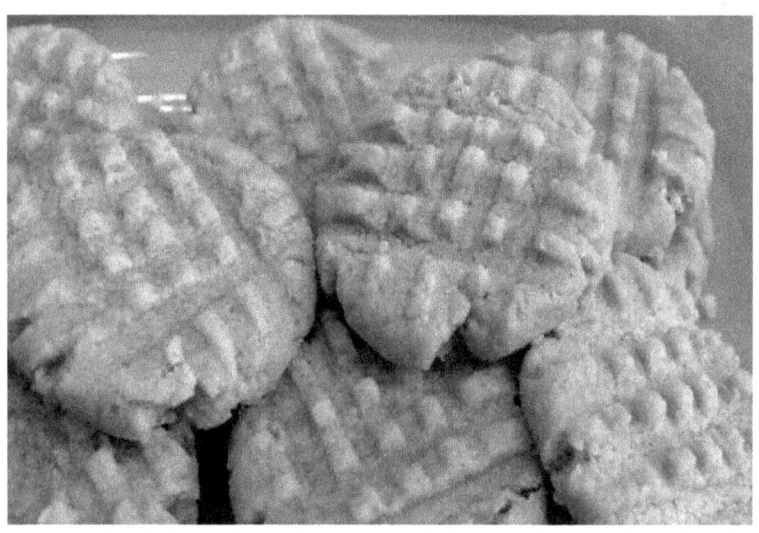

Preparation Time: 10 Minutes

Cooking Time: 15 Minutes

Efforts: Easy

Servings: Makes 12 Cookies

Nutritional Information per serving:
Calories: 140cal, Carbohydrates: 2.8g, Proteins: 5.8g, Fat: 10.4g, Sodium: 134mg

Ingredients:
- ½ tsp. Vanilla Extract
- 1 cup Peanut Butter, smooth
- ½ tsp. Baking Soda
- 1 Egg, large
- 2/3 cup Erythritol, or any low carb sweetener of your choice

Instructions:
1. Preheat the oven to 350°F.
2. Place the erythritol to a blender and blend until powdered.
3. Stir in all the remaining ingredients to the blender and blend until you get a smooth dough.
4. Take two tablespoons of the dough and make it into balls. Repeat with the remaining dough.
5. Place them on a greased parchment paper-lined baking sheet and flatten them slightly with a fork to create a criss-cross pattern while leaving ample space between them.
6. Cook them for 15 minutes or until they are golden brown in colour.
7. Allow it to cool for 28 minutes before serving.

Tip: If you prefer, you can add sugar-free chocolate chips into it.

CHOCOLATE KETO BOMBS

Less than 5 ingredient, Keto & No-cook

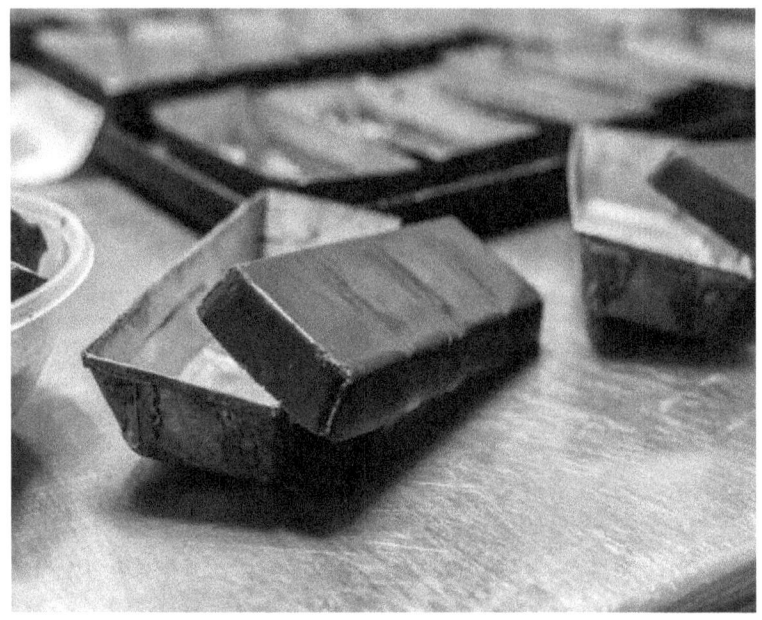

Preparation Time: 5 Minutes

Cooking Time: 5 Minutes

Efforts: Easy

Servings: Makes 6

Nutritional Information per serving:
Calories: 84cal, Carbohydrates: 1.6g, Proteins: 2g, Fat: 8.2g, Sodium: 0mg

Ingredients:

- ½ cup Nut Butter of your choice
- 1 tbsp. Stevia
- ¼ cup Cocoa Powder
- ¼ cup Coconut Oil, melted
- 1/8 tsp. Salt

Instructions:

1. Combine all the ingredients in a medium-sized mixing bowl until mixed well.
2. Transfer the batter to molds or containers or ice cube trays.
3. Place them in the freezer until set.

Tip: Instead of cocoa powder, you can also use cacao powder.

LOW-CARB CHEESECAKE

Less than 5 –ingredients, Nuts-Free & Keto

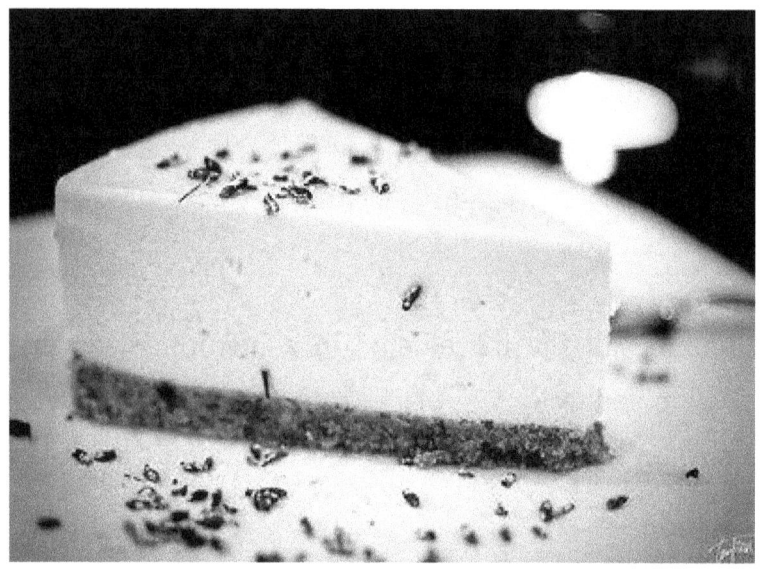

Preparation Time: 10 Minutes

Cooking Time: 50 Minutes

Efforts: Medium

Servings: Makes 12

Nutritional Information per serving:
Calories: 600cal, Carbohydrates: 7g, Proteins: 14g,

Fat: 54g, Sodium: 112mg

Ingredients:

- 6 × 8 oz. Cream Cheese
- 1 tbsp. Vanilla Extract
- 2 cups Sweetener, powdered
- 8 oz. Sour Cream
- 5 Eggs, large & room temperature

Instructions:

1. Check all the ingredients are at room temperature. Then place the cream cheese in a large mixing bowl.
2. Beat it with a hand mixer until it becomes light and fluffy.
3. Add 1/3 of the sweetener at a time to the mixture and continue whisking.
4. Once all the sweetener has been added, stir in the eggs, one at a time.
5. Combine the whole mixture until everything comes together.
6. Spoon in the vanilla extract and mix well.
7. Transfer the mixture to a well-greased parchment paper lined springform pan.
8. Bake them for 50 minutes or until set.
9. Allow the cheesecake to sit for another half hour and then serve.

Tip: You can also make the cheesecake with a crust.

CHOCOLATE AVOCADO PUDDING

Keto, Diary-Free, Nut-Free & Under 30 Minutes

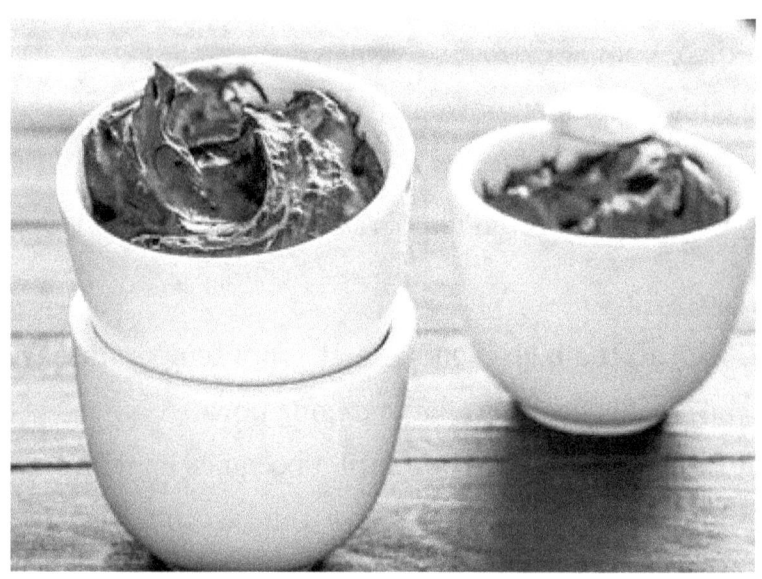

Preparation Time: 10 Minutes

Cooking Time: 10 Minutes

Efforts: Easy

Servings: 6

Nutritional Information per serving:
Calories: 199cal, Carbohydrates: 3.6g, Proteins: 2.9g, Fat: 17.8g, Sodium: 106mg

Ingredients:

- ¼ tsp. Salt
- 2 Avocado, ripe
- 1 tsp. Vanilla Extract
- 1/3 cup Cocoa Powder, unsweetened
- 2/3 cup Coconut Milk
- 1/3 cup Sugar-free Sweetener, powdered

Instructions:

1. Scoop out the avocado flesh and transfer to a blender.
2. Add the remaining ingredients and blend the mixture for a minute.
3. Scrape out the sides and blend further for another 20 to 30 seconds until you get a smooth and luscious mixture.
4. Transfer to the serving jar and place it in the refrigerator for a minimum of at least 1 hour.

Tip: You can make it with a liquid texture, by adding 1 tablespoon of the coconut milk at a time.

RASPBERRY ICE CREAM

Keto, Nuts-Free & Less than 5 ingredients

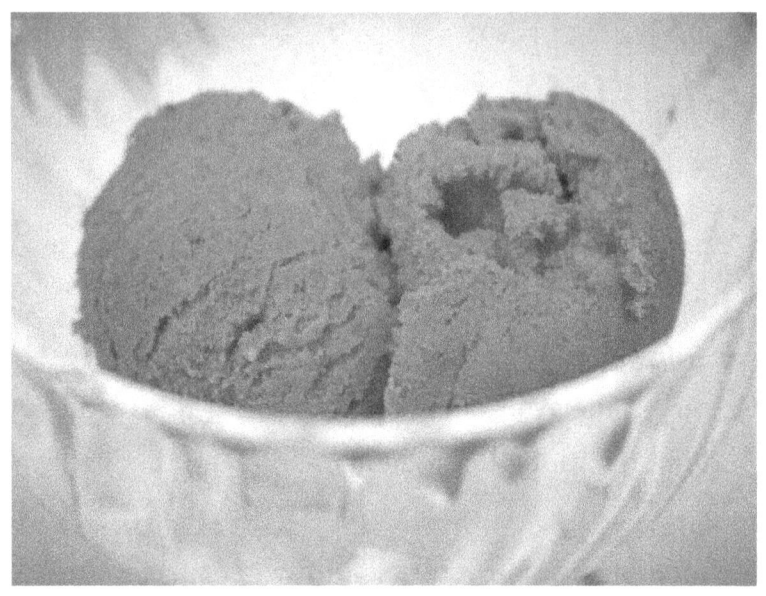

Preparation Time: 5 Minutes

Cooking Time: 5 Minutes

Efforts: Easy

Servings: Makes 5 ½ cups

Nutritional Information per serving:

Calories: 183cal, Carbohydrates: 3g, Proteins: 1g,

Fat: 16g, Sodium: 10mg

Ingredients:
- 1 cup Heavy Cream
- 1/3 cup Erythritol, powdered
- 2 cups Raspberry, frozen

Instructions:
1. Place the heavy cream in a blender and blend for a few minutes or until you get stiff peaks.
2. Stir in the raspberries and erythritol and blend for 3 minutes or until you get a pureed and smooth mixture.
3. Serve and enjoy.

Tip: For firmer ice cream, keep it in the freezer and stir every half to one hour for the first 4 to 5 hours to break ice crystals.

COOKIE DOUGH

Keto & Less than 5 ingredients

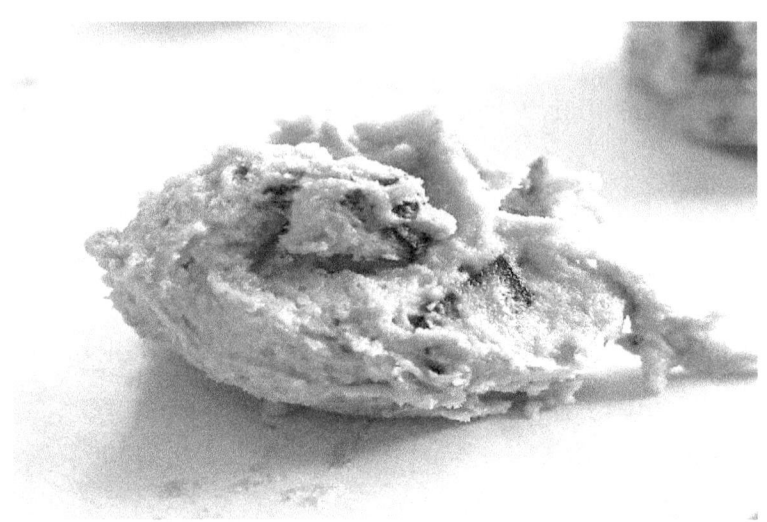

Preparation Time: 5 Minutes

Cooking Time: 5 Minutes

Efforts: Easy

Servings: Makes 14

Nutritional Information per serving:
Calories: 74cal, Carbohydrates: 3g, Proteins: 1.9g, Fat: 6.9g, Sodium: 1.6mg

Ingredients:
- 1 cup Almond Flour
- ¼ cup Sugar-Free Chocolate Chips
- ¼ cup Double Cream
- 1 tbsp. Sweetener, powdered
- ½ tsp. Vanilla Extract

Instructions:
1. Mix all the ingredients in a large mixing bowl. Tip: Add the chocolate chips last in the order.
2. Taste for sweetness and spoon in more if needed.
3. Make balls out of the dough.
4. Serve and enjoy.

Tip: If desired, you can drizzle chocolate ganache syrup over it.

KETO BROWNIES

Less than 30 Minutes

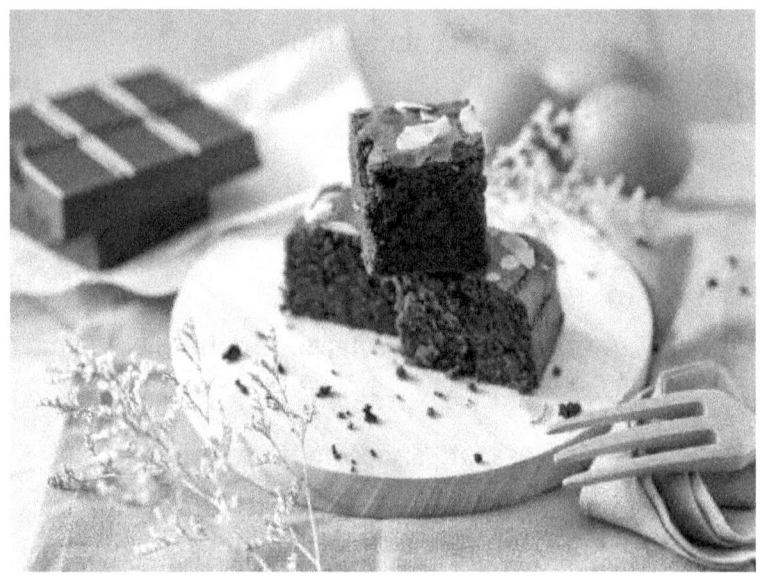

Preparation Time: 10 Minutes

Cooking Time: 20 Minutes

Efforts: Easy

Servings: Makes 14

Nutritional Information per serving:

Calories: 116cal, Carbohydrates: 3g, Proteins: 2g,

Fat: 11g, Sodium: 71mg

Ingredients:
- ½ cup Almond Flour
- 3 Eggs, medium
- ¼ cup Cocoa Powder
- ½ tsp. Baking Powder
- 2 oz. Dark Chocolate
- ¾ cup Erythritol
- 10 tbsp. Butter
- ½ tsp. Vanilla Extract

Instructions:
1. Preheat the oven to 350° F.
2. Combine almond flour, erythritol, cocoa powder, and baking powder in a medium-sized mixing bowl with a whisker.
3. Place butter and chocolate in a microwave-safe bowl and melt for 30 seconds to 1 minute or until melted.
4. Stir in eggs and vanilla to the mixture until mixed well.
5. Once combined, spoon in the dry ingredients and whisk until mixed.
6. Pour the mixture to a greased baking dish and bake for 19 minutes or until a sharp tool comes clean.
7. Allow it to cool for 2 hours in the refrigerator and serve.

Tip: If preferred, you can stir in chocolate chips or chopped chocolate into it.

KEY LIME PIE

Keto

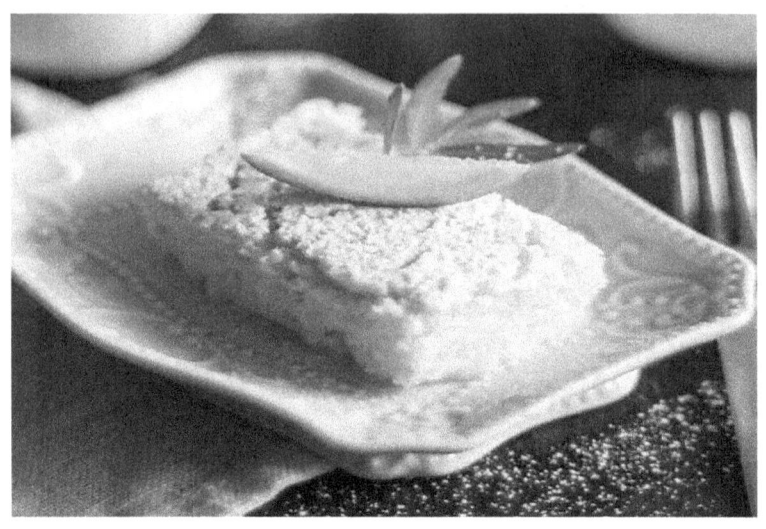

Preparation Time: 15 Minutes

Cooking Time: 1 Hour

Efforts: Easy

Servings: Makes 16 slices

Nutritional Information per serving:

Calories: 325cal, Carbohydrates: 5g, Proteins: 4g,

Fat: 32g, Sodium: 21mg

Ingredients:
For the base:

- 3 oz. Butter, melted
- 7 oz. Almond Meal
- 1 tbsp. Swerve
- ¼ cup Golden Flax Meal

For the filling:
- Zest of 3 Limes
- ½ cup Heavy Cream
- 4 Eggs
- 14 oz. Condensed Milk, sugar-free
- ½ cup Key Lime Juice

For topping:
- 7 fl. oz. Heavy Cream

Instructions:
1. Preheat the oven to 340° F.
2. Mix almond meal, swerve, and flax meal in a large mixing bowl until combined.
3. Spoon in the melted butter and stir.
4. Transfer the mixture to a greased springform pan and press it slightly down and up the sides.
5. Bake for 12 minutes. Allow it to cool.

To make the filling
1. Lower the temperature to 300°F.
2. Whisk egg and condensed milk in another bowl on medium speed and slowly lower the speed.
3. Pour the lime juice slowly to it, followed by cream and lime zest.
4. Transfer the mixture onto the top of the crust and bake for further 40 minutes or until just set in the center.
5. Allow it to cool for 20 minutes and then place in the refrigerator for 2 hours.
6. Whip the cream and spread.
7. Serve and enjoy.

Tip: Top it with whipped cream and nuts if desired.

KETO VANILLA MUG CAKE

Nuts-Free & Less than 30 Minutes

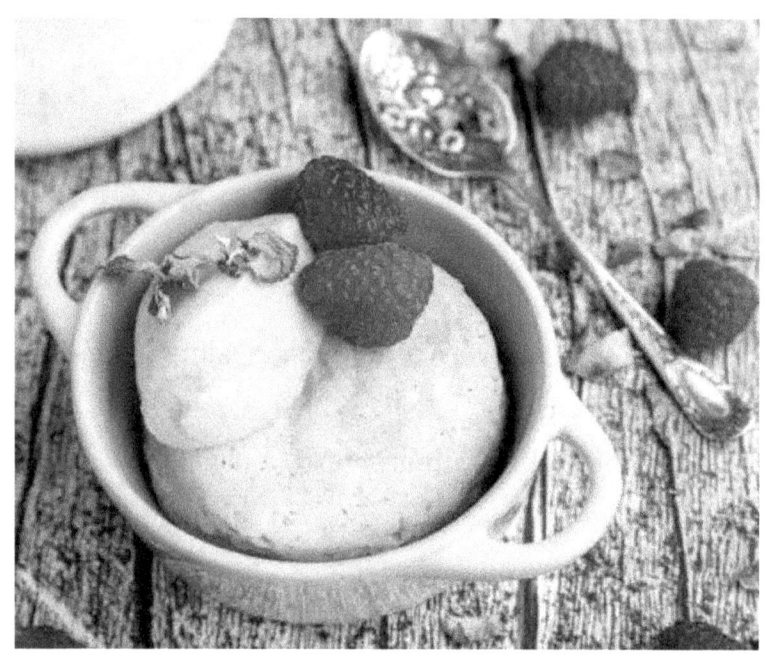

Preparation Time: 5 Minutes

Cooking Time: 1 Minute

Efforts: Easy

Servings: 1

Nutritional Information per serving:
Calories: 342cal, Carbohydrates: 4.5g, Proteins: 9g, Fat: 27g, Sodium: 17mg

Ingredients:

- ¼ tsp. Baking Powder
- 1 tbsp. Butter, melted
- 1 tsp. Vanilla Extract
- 2 tbsp. Cream Cheese
- 1 Egg
- 2 tbsp. Coconut Flour
- 6 Raspberries, frozen
- 1 tbsp. Low-Carb Sweetener, granulated

Instructions:

1. Place butter and cream cheese in a large mug and heat on high power for 20 seconds.
2. Spoon in coconut flour, baking powder, sweetener, and vanilla to it. Combine.
3. Add the egg to it and stir it again.
4. Scrape down the sides and press the six raspberries to it.
5. Heat the batter again for 1 minute and 20 seconds on high power.
6. Allow it to cool and set aside.

Tip: If you want a simple vanilla cake, you can avoid the raspberries.

LEMON COOKIES

Keto & Under 30 Minutes

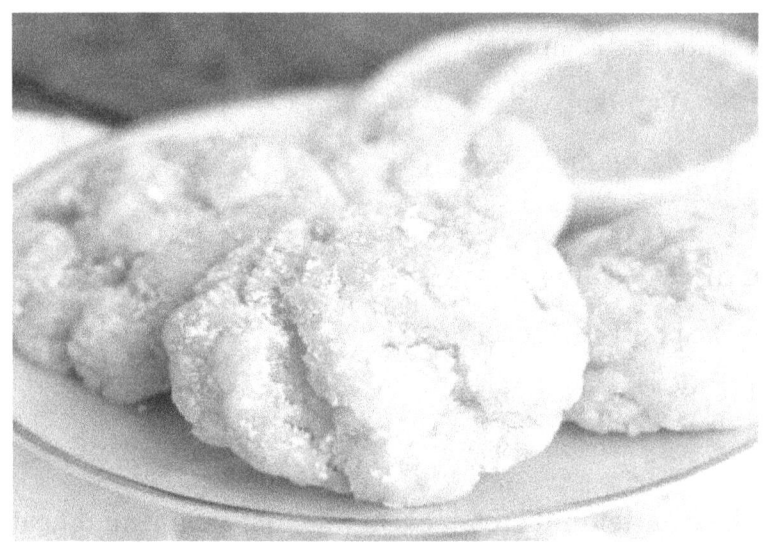

Preparation Time: 5 Minutes

Cooking Time: 20 Minutes

Efforts: Easy

Servings: Makes 12

Nutritional Information per serving:

Calories: 150cal, Carbohydrates: 4.5g, Proteins: 9g,

Fat: 27g, Sodium: 17mg

Ingredients:
- ¼ cup Cream Cheese
- Zest of 1 Lemon
- ¼ cup Butter, unsalted
- 4 tbsp. Lemon Juice

- 5 tbsp. Erythritol, powdered
- 2 cup Almond Flour
- 1 Egg, medium

For the glaze:
- ¼ cup Erythritol, powdered
- Lemon Zest, as needed
- 1 ½ tbsp. Lemon Juice

Instructions:

1. Place cream cheese, lemon zest, butter, and four tablespoon lemon juice in a food processor and process until smooth.
2. Stir in the egg and combine.
3. Once it is combined, add the almond flour and mix again.
4. Wrap the soft dough in a cling wrap and place in the refrigerator for 20 to 25 minutes.
5. Preheat the oven to 356° F.
6. Make balls out of the dough and arrange them on a parchment-paper-lined baking tray while making sure to flatten the balls slightly.
7. Bake them for 10 to 15 minutes or until lightly browned at the bottom.
8. Allow it to cool while making the glaze by mixing erythritol, lemon zest, and lemon juice. Spoon the lemon glaze over the cooled cookies and serve.

Tip: If you want a simple vanilla cake, you can avoid the raspberries.

CHIA PUDDING

Keto, Diary-Free & Less than 5 Ingredients

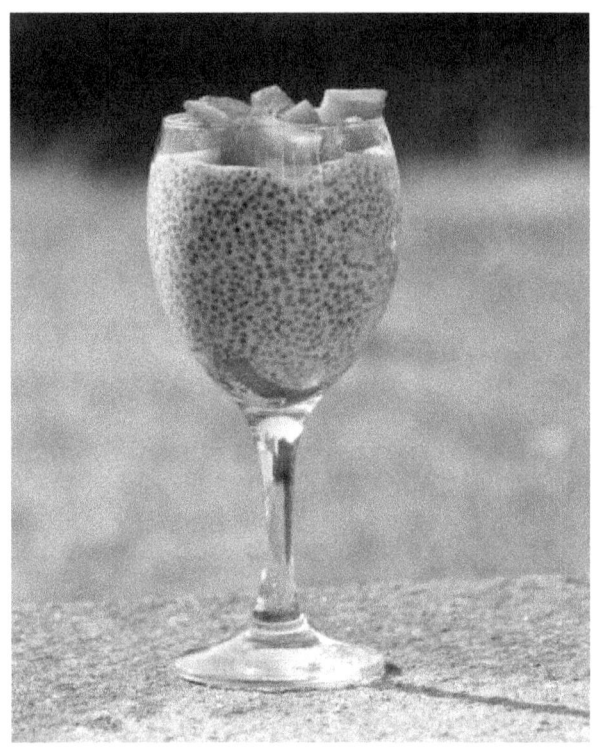

Preparation Time: 10 Minutes

Cooking Time: 0 Minutes

Efforts: Easy

Servings: 1

Nutritional Information per serving:
Calories: 151cal, Carbohydrates: 1.5g, Proteins: 5g,

Fat: 10g, Sodium: 328mg

Ingredients:
- 2 tbsp. Chia Seeds
- 1 cup Almond Milk
- 1 tsp. Stevia, vanilla flavoured

Instructions:

1. Mix the chia seeds and almond milk thoroughly until combined well.
2. Set it aside for overnight in the refrigerator.
3. Serve and enjoy. You can top with topping of your choice like berries, nuts, etc.

Tip: If desired, you can add more liquid and sweetener according to your choice.

STRAWBERRY POPSICLES

Keto & Less than 5 Ingredient

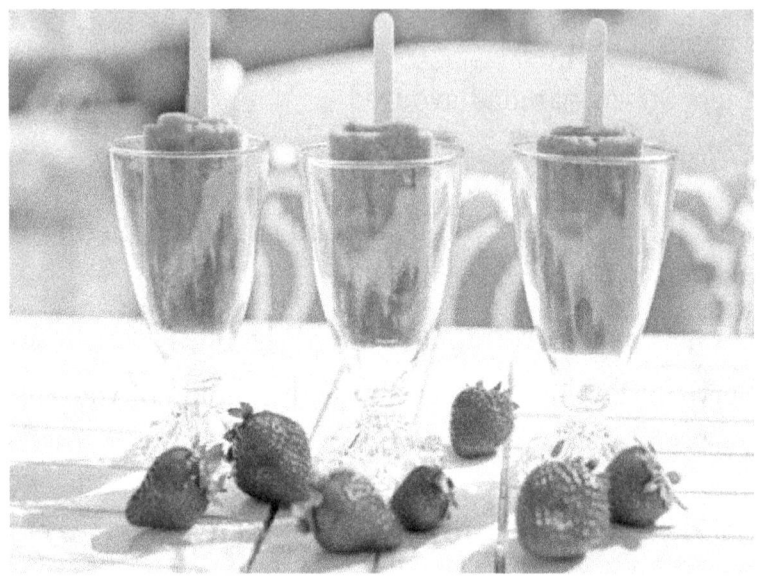

Preparation Time: 5 Minutes

Cooking Time: 0 Minutes + 3 Hours Cooling Time

Efforts: Easy

Servings: 6

Nutritional Information per serving:
Calories: 73cal, Carbohydrates: 12g, Proteins: 3.5g,

Fat: 0.5g, Sodium: 67mg

Ingredients:

- 5 drops of Liquid Stevia
- ¼ cup Oats, old-fashioned, grounded
- 4 oz. Cottage Cheese, low-fat
- Juice from 4 Lemons
- 1 ½ lb. Strawberries

Instructions:

1. Add all the ingredients in a high-speed blender and blend until it becomes smooth.
2. Once pureed, pour the mixture to the popsicle molds and place it in the freezer overnight or for a minimum of 6 hours.
3. Serve and enjoy.

Tip: Meyer's lemon would be the best choice to use for lemons.

CHOLATE FUDGE

Keto

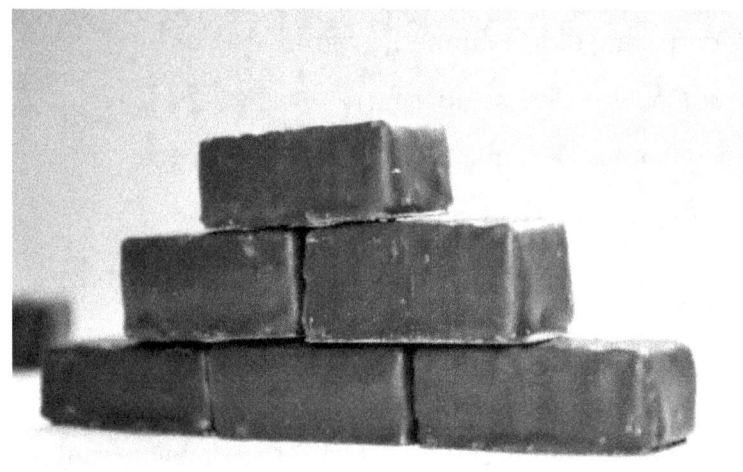

Preparation Time: 15 Minutes

Cooking Time: 15 Minutes

Efforts: Easy

Servings: Makes 12 Fudges

Nutritional Information per serving:
Calories: 154.77cal, Carbohydrates: 10.79g, Proteins: 1.87g,

Fat: 15.5g, Sodium: 29mg

Ingredients:
- ¼ cup Pecans, chopped
- 1 cup Heavy Whipping Cream
- 1 cup Chocolate Chips, low-carb
- 1/3 cup Erythritol
- 1 tsp. Vanilla Extract
- 2 tbsp. Butter

Instructions:
1. Heat a medium-sized pan and to this, stir in whipping cream, vanilla extract, butter, and erythritol.
2. Continue stirring for 15 minutes or until you get a slightly browned condensed milk with a thick texture.
3. Allow to cool for 12 minutes and then add the chocolate chips.
4. Once the chocolate chips have melted, pour the mixture to a parchment paper-lined loaf pan and top it with pecans.
5. Keep in the refrigerator for at least an hour or more.
6. Serve and enjoy.

Tip: Instead of pecans, you can use any pecans.

CHOCOLATE MOUSSE

Keto, Less than 5 ingredients & Under 30 Minutes

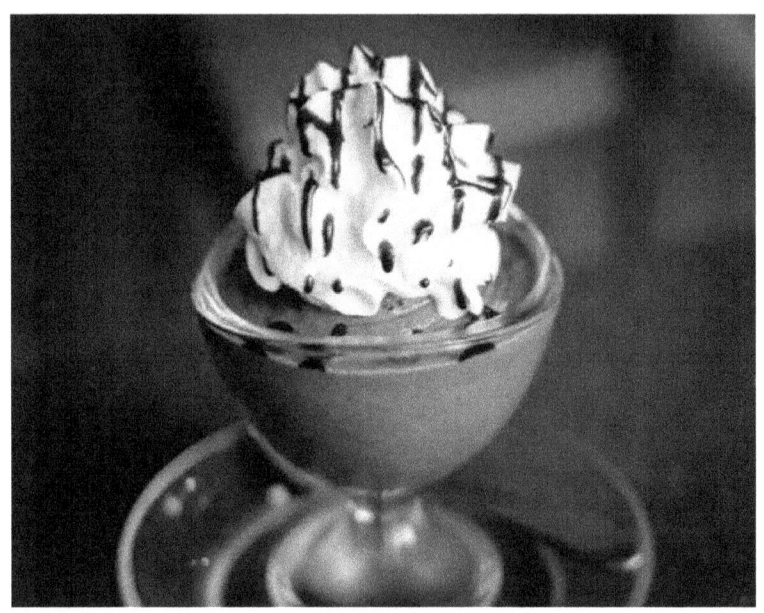

Preparation Time: 10 Minutes

Cooking Time: 5 Minutes

Efforts: Easy

Servings: 4

Nutritional Information per serving:

Calories: 218cal, Carbohydrates: 3g, Proteins: 2g,

Fat: 23g, Sodium: 29mg

Ingredients:
- 1/4 cup Cocoa Powder, unsweetened
- 1 cup Heavy Whipping Cream
- 1 tsp. Vanilla Extract
- ¼ cup Low-Carb Sweetener, powdered
- ¼ tsp. Salt

Instructions:

1. Place the whipping cream in a large mixing bowl and whisk it with a mixer until you get stiff peaks.
2. Stir in the remaining ingredients and whisk until everything comes together.
3. Serve and enjoy.

Tip: If you prefer a lighter texture mousse, add three egg whites and whisk them to stiff peaks before mixing in.

CHOCOLATE COCONUT BALLSKETO

Diary-Free & Less than 30 Minutes

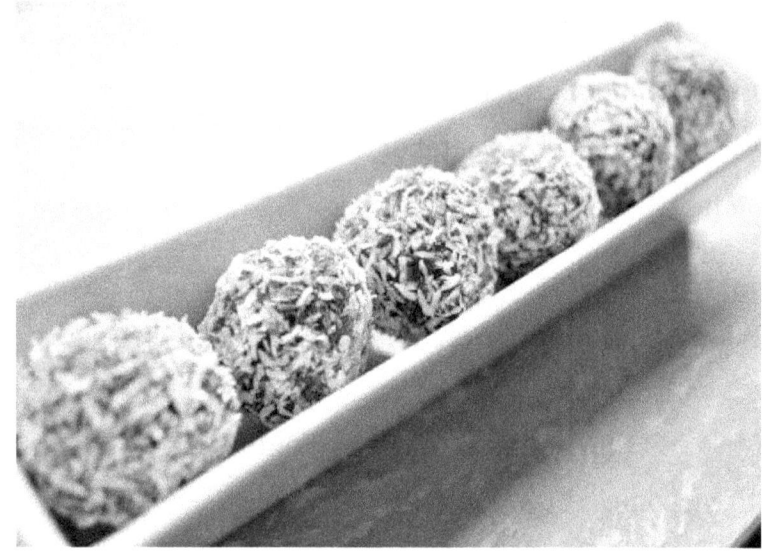

Preparation Time: 10 Minutes

Cooking Time: 5 Minutes

Efforts: Easy

Servings: Makes 14 Balls

Nutritional Information per serving:
Calories: 134cal, Carbohydrates: 21g, Proteins: 2g,

Fat: 7g, Sodium: 34mg

Ingredients:

- 1 tsp. Vanilla Extract
- 9 Dates, pitted
- 1 ¼ cup Coconut Flakes, shredded & unsweetened
- 1 Banana, mashed
- 4 tbsp. Cocoa Powder
- ½ tsp. Liquid Stevia, chocolate
- ¼ tsp. Salt
- ½ cup Chocolate Chips, sugar-free

Instructions:

1. Place banana, one cup of the coconut flakes, and cocoa in a food processor. Blend for a minute or so.
2. Stir in the dates, chopped, bit by bit into it and blend again.
3. Spoon in the stevia, salt, and vanilla extract to it and stir again.
4. Transfer the mixture to a large-sized mixing bowl and add the chocolate chips to it.
5. Place ¼ of the remaining coconut flakes to a large plate.
6. Make balls out of the mixture and roll them in the coconut flakes until coated well.
7. Finally, keep in the refrigerator until served.
8. Serve and enjoy.

Tip: Instead of chocolate chips, you could use nuts of your choice also.

VANILLA BEAN ICE CREAM

Keto & Less than 5 ingredients

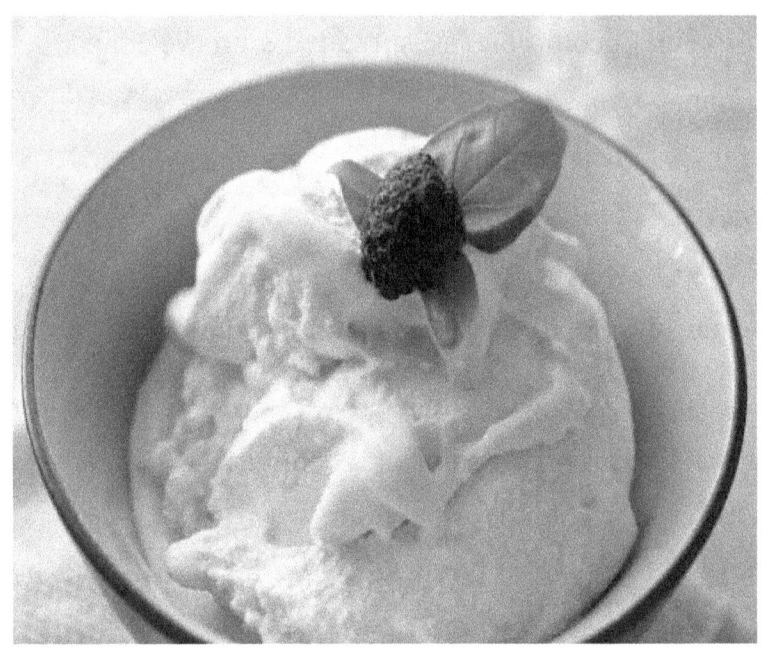

Preparation Time: 10 Minutes

Cooking Time: 10 Minutes

Efforts: Easy

Servings: 1

Nutritional Information per serving:
Calories: 172cal, Carbohydrates: 5.2g, Proteins: 4.1g,

Fat: 15.2g, Sodium: 140mg

Ingredients:
- ½ cup Half & Half
- 4 drops of Vanilla Liquid Stevia
- ½ cup Almond Milk, vanilla flavoured & unsweetened
- Dash of Salt
- ½ of 1 Vanilla Bean Pod or ½ tsp. Vanilla Extract

Instructions:
1. Place half & half and almond milk to the blender.
2. Slice the vanilla pod into two center wise into it along with the remaining ingredients.
3. Blend for a minute or two and then transfer the mixture to an ice cream machine.
4. Serve immediately and enjoy it.

Tip: You can top it with chocolate sauce.

CHOCOLATE ZUCCHINI CAKE

Keto & Diary-Free

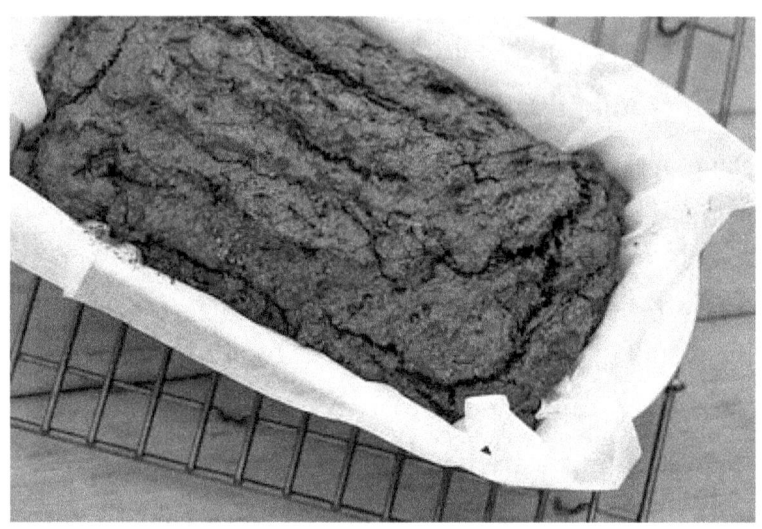

Preparation Time: 15 Minutes

Cooking Time: 1 Hour

Efforts: Easy

Servings: Makes 10 slices

Nutritional Information per serving:
Calories: 265cal, Carbohydrates: 8.5g, Proteins: 8.72g,

Fat: 23.6g, Sodium: 27mg

Ingredients:
- ¼ cup Cocoa Powder
- 1 cup Sukrin Gold
- 2 cups Almond Flour, blanched
- ½ tsp. Baking Soda
- 1 tbsp. Espresso Powder
- 1 tsp. Baking Powder
- ½ cup Chocolate Chips, sugar-free

For the wet ingredients:

- 1 Zucchini
- 3 Eggs, medium
- 1 tbsp. Apple Cider Vinegar
- ¼ cup Refined Coconut Oil
- ¼ cup Almond Milk, unsweetened

Instructions:
1. Preheat the oven to 350° F.
2. Shred the zucchini and place it in the cheesecloth and squeeze out all the water.
3. Keep the zucchini in a large mixing bowl and, to this, stir in all the dry ingredients. Combine well.
4. Add all the wet ingredients to it one by one and give everything a good stir.
5. Transfer the batter to an oiled baking pan and bake for 60 minutes or until cooked.
6. Allow it to cool and enjoy.

Tip: You can top it with chocolate sauce.

CHOCOLATE PEANUT BUTTER BLONDIES

Keto & Diary-Free

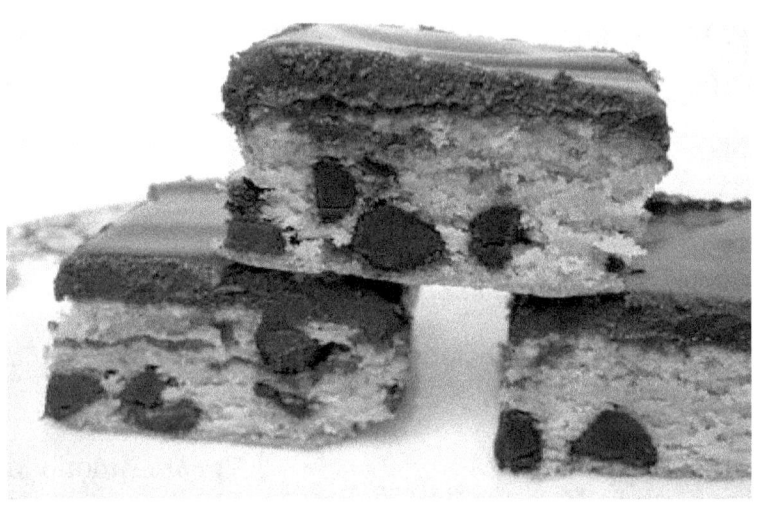

Preparation Time: 15 Minutes

Cooking Time: 1 Hour

Efforts: Easy

Servings: Makes 10 slices

Nutritional Information per serving:
Calories: 265cal, Carbohydrates: 8.5g, Proteins: 8.72g, Fat: 23.6g, Sodium: 27mg

Ingredients:
- 1 ½ cup Chickpeas
- 1 tsp. Baking Powder
- 1 Egg
- ½ cup Peanut Butter, unsweetened
- ¼ cup Coconut Oil

- ½ cup Erythritol
- 1 tsp. Liquid Stevia, vanilla
- ¼ tsp. Salt
- ½ tsp. Vanilla Extract

For the chocolate layer:

- 3 tbsp. Erythritol
- ½ cup Cocoa Powder, unsweetened
- 4 tbsp. Coconut Oil

Instructions:

1. Preheat the oven to 350° F.
2. Mix all the ingredients, excluding the chocolate layer into the food processor and process until blended.
3. Transfer the peanut butter layer to a parchment paper-lined baking pan and spread it out evenly.
4. Make the chocolate layer by placing the coconut oil in a microwave-safe bowl and heat for 20 seconds or until melted.
5. Once melted, stir in the cocoa powder and erythritol and whisk well.
6. Spoon the chocolate layer gradually over the peanut butter layer and bake for 25 to 30 minutes.
7. Take off the pan from the oven and set it aside for 30 minutes.
8. Enjoy.

Tip: Instead of erythritol, you can also use applesauce or honey.

BOUNTY BARS

Keto & Diary-Free

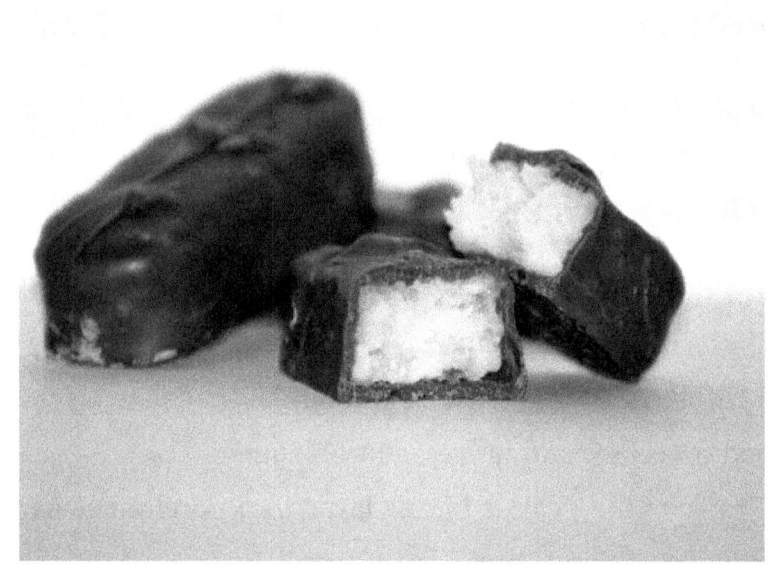

Preparation Time: 10 Minutes

Cooking Time: 30 Minutes

Efforts: Easy

Servings: 20

Nutritional Information per serving:
Calories: 100cal, Carbohydrates: 6g, Proteins: 0.5g,

Fat: 7.3g, Sodium: 23mg

Ingredients:
- 1/3 cup Erythritol
- 2 cups Desiccated Coconut, unsweetened
- 1/3 cup Coconut Oil
- ½ cup Coconut Cream

For the chocolate layer:

- 6 oz. Chocolate Chips, sugar-free
- 2 tsp. Coconut Oil

Instructions:
1. Cover a square baking pan with plastic wrap.
2. Place all the ingredients needed to make the filling in a food processor, excluding the ones required for the chocolate layer.
3. Process it until you get a dough.
4. Place the dough onto the prepared pan and spread it across evenly while making sure no air left between the dough.
5. Place the pan in the freezer for 10 minutes.
6. Once ten minutes has past, take out the plastic wrap from the pan to release the coconut bar quickly.
7. With the aid of a knife, slice the coconut layers into 20 bars.
8. In the meantime, melt the coconut oil and chocolate chips in a microwave-safe bowl for 20 seconds on high power.
9. Using two forks, dip the coconut bars into the melted chocolate mixture until coated fully.
10. Place the bars onto a rack and freeze them again for further 10 minutes.
11. Serve and enjoy.

Tip: If preferred, you can add liquid stevia to the chocolate layer for more sweetness.

CHOCOLATE ICE CREAM

Keto

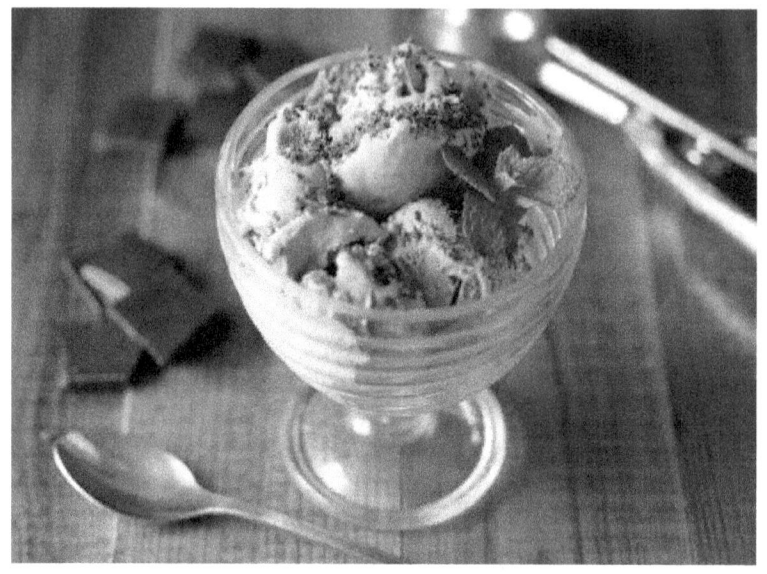

Preparation Time: 10 Minutes

Cooking Time: 0 + 2 Hours Setting Time

Efforts: Easy

Servings: 1 to 2

Nutritional Information per serving:
Calories: 127cal, Carbohydrates: 5.6g, Proteins: 20.1g,

Fat: 2.2g, Sodium: 150m

Ingredients:

- ½ cup Almond Milk, unsweetened
- 2 ½ oz. Greek Yoghurt, fat-free
- 2 tbsp. Stevia
- ½ oz. Protein Powder
- 1 tsp. Vanilla Extract
- 1 tsp. Cocoa Powder, unsweetened

Instructions:

1. Place yogurt, almond milk, cocoa powder, stevia, and protein powder in a high-speed blender.
2. Blend them for few minutes or until you get a smooth mixture.
3. Place in the freezer to set.
4. Take out the ice cream every 30 seconds and blend. Repeat the procedure for about 2 hours until you get the right consistency without any ice blocks.
5. Serve and enjoy.

Tip: If desired, you can top it with nuts or berries.

3.6 EXTRA RECIPES

BREAKFAST

QUINOA PORRIDGE

Less than 30 Min & Under 5 ingredients

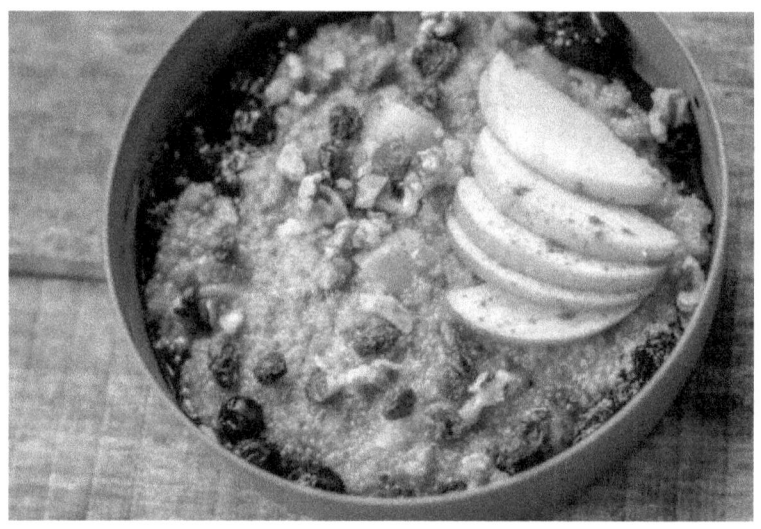

Preparation Time: 5 Minutes

Cooking Time: 5 Minutes

Efforts: Easy

Servings: 1

Nutritional Information per serving:
Calories: 159Kcal, Carbohydrates: 23.6g, Proteins: 18.1g, Fat: 5.3g, Sodium: 284mg

Ingredients:
- ½ cup Quinoa, dry, washed & drained
- 1 cup Water
- 1/3 cup low-carb fruit of your choice, chopped
- ½ to 1 cup Milk of your choice
- Low-carb Sweeteners of your choice, as needed

Instructions:
1. Keep the quinoa and water in a medium-sized saucepan and heat it over medium-high heat.
2. Bring the mixture to a boil and allow it to gently simmer for 10 to 12 minutes or until the quinoa is cooked and all the water has absorbed.
3. Remove the pan from the heat and allow it to cool. Once cooled, fluff it with a fork.
4. Mix the quinoa with the milk. Stir well.
5. Finally, add fruits and sweetener to it. Mix.
6. Serve and enjoy.

Tip: You can even spice of your choice like cinnamon for more flavor.

OATMEAL WITH SWEET POTATOES

Under 30 Minutes

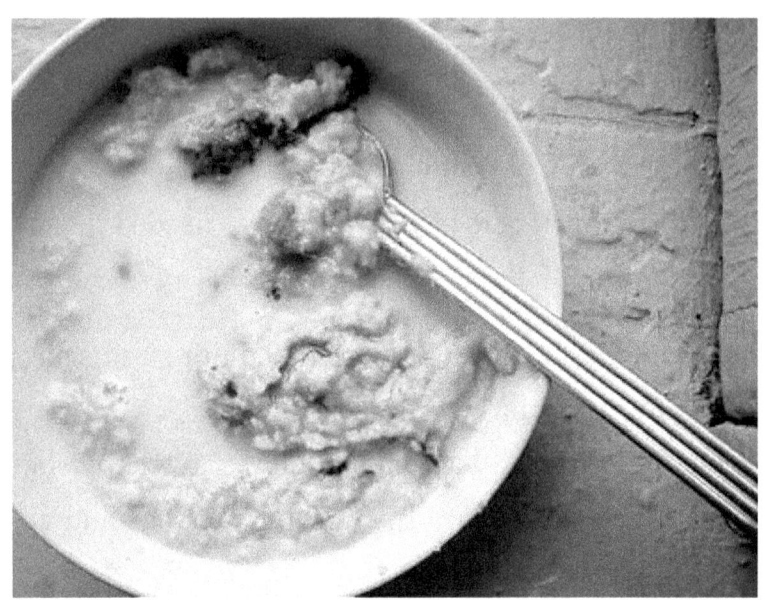

Preparation Time: 5 Minutes

Cooking Time: 5 Minutes

Efforts: Easy

Servings: 1

Nutritional Information per serving:
Calories: 200Kcal, Carbohydrates: 18.7g, Proteins: 7.6g,
Fat: 9.8g, Sodium: 158mg

Ingredients:
- ½ cup Oatmeal
- 1 tsp. Coconut Sugar or Turbinado Sugar
- 2/3 cup Milk of your choice
- Low-carb sweetener of your choice, as needed
- Dash of Salt
- ½ tsp. Pumpkin Pie Spice
- 1/3 cup Sweet Potato, mashed
- 2 to 3 tbsp. Almonds, chopped

Instructions:

1. Combine oats, mashed sweet potato, milk, and salt in a microwave-safe bowl. Heat it for 1 to 1 ½ minute at high power.
2. Take out the bowl and spoon in the low-carb sweetener and pumpkin pie spice to it. Mix well.
3. Serve warm.

Tip: You can add low-sugar maple syrup if desired.

BANANA EGG OATMEAL

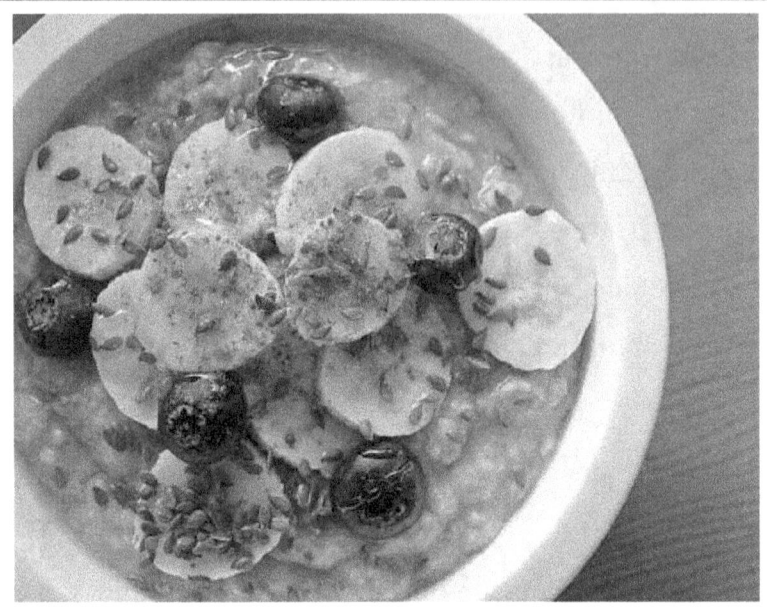

Preparation Time: 5 Minutes

Cooking Time: 5 Minutes

Efforts: Easy

Servings: 1 to 2

Nutritional Information per serving:
Calories: 200Kcal, Carbohydrates: 18.7g, Proteins: 7.6g,

Fat: 9.8g, Sodium: 158mg

Ingredients:
- Dash of Cinnamon
- 1/3 cup Oats
- Pinch of Salt
- 2/3 cup Water
- 1/8 tsp. Vanilla Extract
- ½ of 1 Banana, mashed
- 1 tbsp. Nuts

Instructions:
1. Place all the ingredients needed to make the oatmeal in a small saucepan over medium heat.
2. Allow the oatmeal to boil and once it starts boiling, continue stirring for 4 minutes or until all the liquid is absorbed.
3. Take the saucepan from the heat. Set it aside for 5 minutes.
4. Serve it warm and top with the nuts.

Tip: You can also top it with berries.

BROILED GRAPEFRUIT

Paleo, Less than 30 Min & Under 5 ingredients

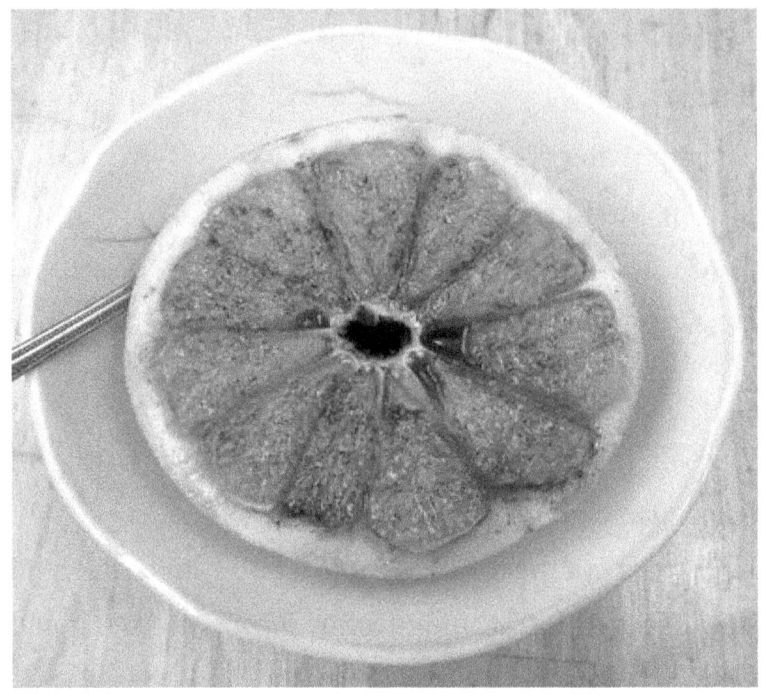

Preparation Time: 5 Minutes

Cooking Time: 5 Minutes

Efforts: Easy

Servings: 4

Nutritional Information per serving:
Calories: 108Kcal, Carbohydrates: 26g, Proteins: 1g,

Fat: 0g, Sodium: 8mg

Ingredients:

- 2 Grapefruit, halved
- Strawberries, as needed
- 1 tbsp. Low-carb sweetener syrup of your choice
- ¼ tsp. Cinnamon, grounded & as needed

Instructions:

1. Preheat the broiler.
2. Place the halved grapefruit on a baking sheet.
3. Spoon the sweetener syrup over each of the halved fruit and dust it with the grounded cinnamon.
4. Broil the grapefruit for 6 minutes or until slightly browned.
5. Serve and enjoy.

Tip: You can also top it with grounded ginger.

NUTS & SEED CEREAL

Less than 30 Minutes & Keto

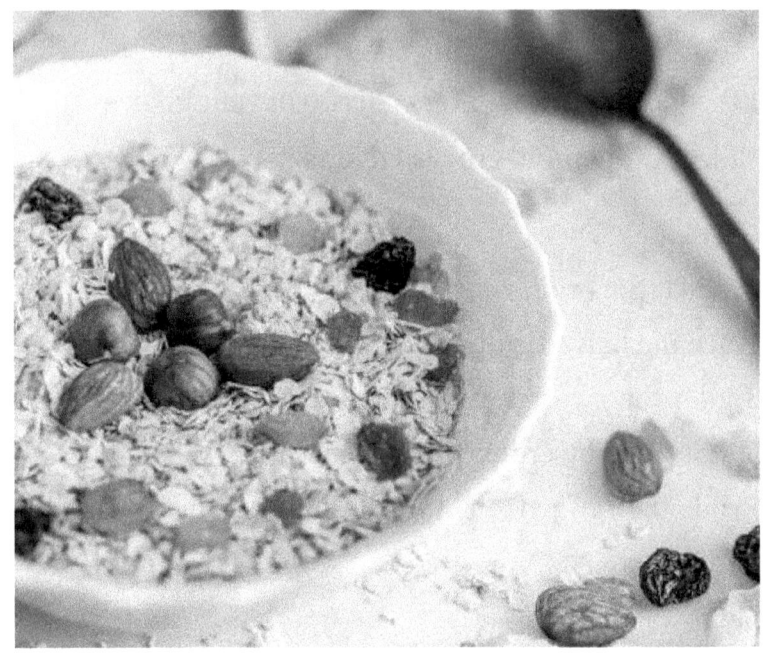

Preparation Time: 10 Minutes

Cooking Time: 0 Minutes

Efforts: Easy

Servings: 2 to 4

Nutritional Information per serving:
Calories: 277Kcal, Carbohydrates: 19.3g, Proteins: 12.3g, Fat: 14.4g, Sodium: 88mg

Ingredients:
- 1 cup Plain Yoghurt
- 2 tbsp. Sesame Seeds
- ½ tsp. Vanilla
- 2 tbsp. Almond Meal
- ½ tsp. Cinnamon
- 2 tbsp. Hazelnut Meal
- 2 tbsp. Flaxseed Meal

Instructions:
1. Place all the ingredients excluding the yogurt in a large mixing bowl until combined well.
2. Then, top it with yogurt.
3. Serve and enjoy.

Tip: You can also top it with fruits like the pear.

ARUGULA SMOOTHIE

Keto & Under 30 Minutes

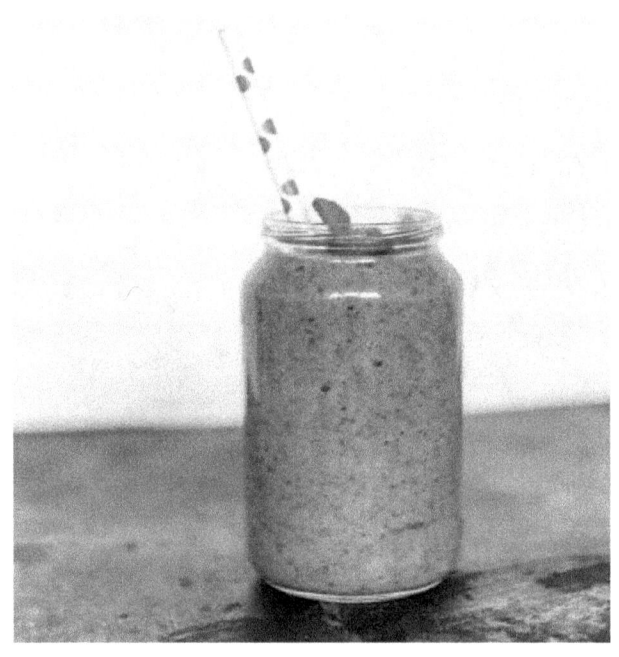

Preparation Time: 10 Minutes

Cooking Time: 0 Minutes

Efforts: Easy

Servings: 2

Nutritional Information per serving:

Calories: 237Kcal, Carbohydrates: 9.8g, Proteins: 12.1g,

Fat: 14.3g, Sodium: 87mg

Ingredients:

- 1 cup Kale
- 1 can of Coconut Milk
- ½ cup Cashew, dry-roasted
- 1 Apple, cored & chopped
- 1 tsp. Cinnamon
- 1-inch piece of Ginger
- 1 cup Arugula
- ½ tsp. Turmeric
- Water, as needed
- ½ tsp. Cinnamon, grounded
- 3 tbsp. Pea Protein Powder

Instructions:

1. Place all the ingredients in a high-speed blender until it becomes smooth, and everything comes together.
2. Serve and enjoy.

Tip: You can also top it flaxseeds if desired.

EGG SCRAMBLE WITH BEANS

Less than 30 Minutes

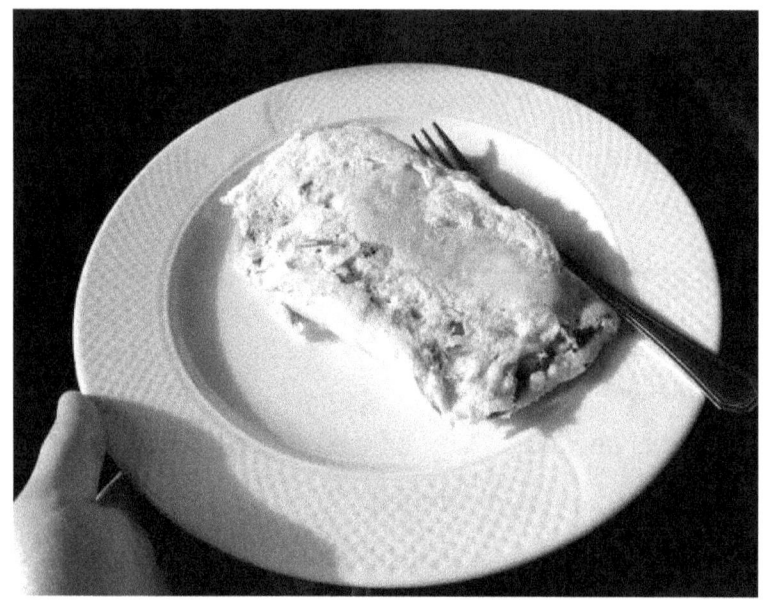

Preparation Time: 10 Minutes

Cooking Time: 5 Minutes

Efforts: Easy

Servings: 2

Nutritional Information per serving:
Calories: 478Kcal, Carbohydrates: 34g, Proteins: 31.5g,

Fat: 15g, Sodium: 144mg

Ingredients:

- 1 Tomato, medium & diced
- ½ tsp. Mexican Spice Seasoning
- 4 Eggs
- 1 Avocado, ripe & chopped
- 15 oz. Black Beans
- 1 cup Spinach, fresh & chopped
- Olive oil, as needed
- ¼ of 1 Onion, diced

Instructions:

1. Place the eggs and Mexican spice in a bowl. Whisk it well and set it aside.
2. Heat olive oil in a large pan over medium heat, and once the oil becomes hot, stir in the onion.
3. Cook for 3 minutes or until softened.
4. Add the beaten eggs to it and cook for further 1 minute or until set.
5. Stir in the spinach and continue cooking until cooked.
6. Transfer the omelet to the plate and top it with avocado.
7. Serve and enjoy.

Tip: You can also top it with salsa.

HERBED CHICKEN SAUSAGE PATTIES

Less than 5 ingredients

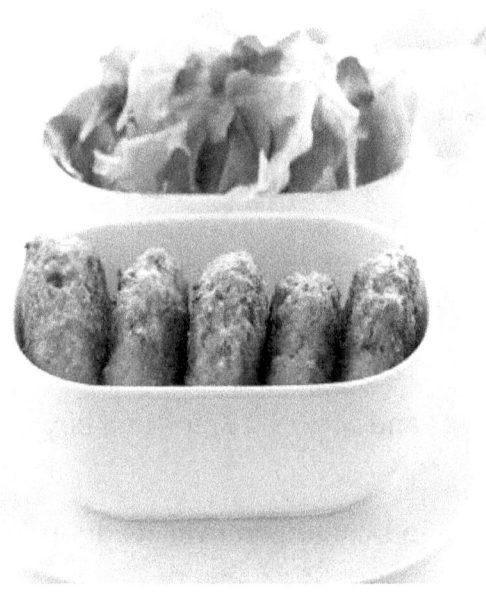

Preparation Time: 15 Minutes

Cooking Time: 20 Minutes

Efforts: Easy

Servings: Makes 8 to 10 patties

Nutritional Information per serving:
Calories: 478Kcal, Carbohydrates: 34g, Proteins: 31.5g,

Fat: 15g, Sodium: 144mg

Ingredients:

- 2 tbsp. Parsley, fresh & chopped
- 1 lb. Turkey, lean & ground
- 1 tbsp. Extra Virgin Olive Oil
- 1 tsp. Poultry Seasoning
- ½ tsp. Sea Salt

Instructions:

1. Preheat the oven to 400° F.
2. Combine turkey, sea salt, olive oil, parsley, and salt in a large mixing bowl with your hands until mixed well.
3. Make 8 to 10 patties out of this meat mixture.
4. Place the patties in a greased baking sheet.
5. Bake them for 19 minutes or until cooked.

Tip: You can serve it with a hearty green salad.

LUNCH

LAMB CHOPS

Keto & Under 30 Minutes

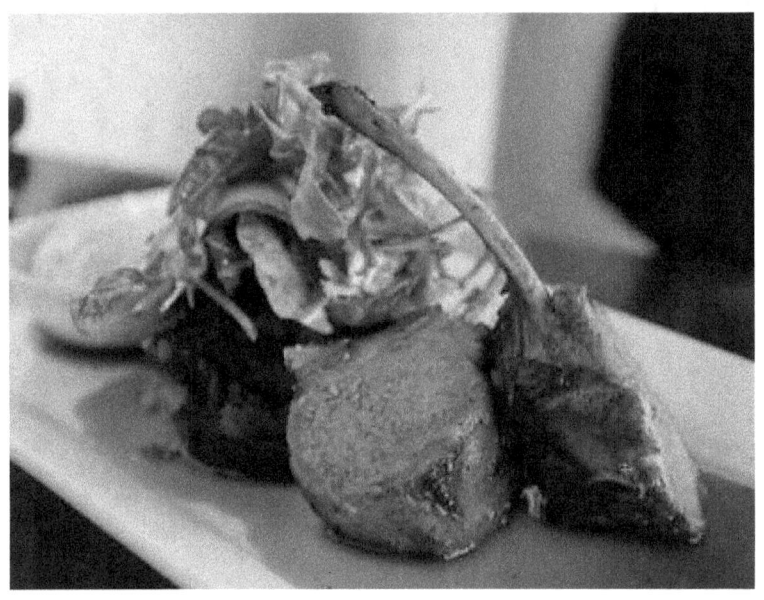

Preparation Time: 5 Minutes

Cooking Time: 10 Minutes

Efforts: Easy

Servings: 4

Nutritional Information per serving:
Calories: 358Kcal, Carbohydrates: 1.2g, Proteins: 46.3g,

Fat: 17.9g, Sodium: 345mg

Ingredients:

- 1 tsp. Pepper
- 2 lb. Lamb Shoulder Chops, washed & pat dry
- 1 tsp. Parsley, dried
- 2 tbsp. Butter
- 4 Garlic cloves, minced
- 1 tsp. Rosemary, dried
- Salt, as needed

Instructions:

1. Combine rosemary, pepper, salt, parsley, and garlic in a small bowl until mixed well.
2. Apply the seasoning mix over the lamb chops and set it aside.
3. Allow the chops to be marinated for a minimum of 30 minutes or a maximum period of 24 hours, if possible.
4. Heat a medium-sized skillet over medium-high heat.
5. Once the skillet is hot, melt the butter.
6. Stir in the chops and cook them for 4 minutes per side or until cooked and browned. Tip: Don't overcrowd the skillet while cooking.
7. Serve hot and enjoy it.

Tip: You can serve it with a green salad or cauliflower rice.

BAKED COD WITH LEMON

Under 30 Minutes

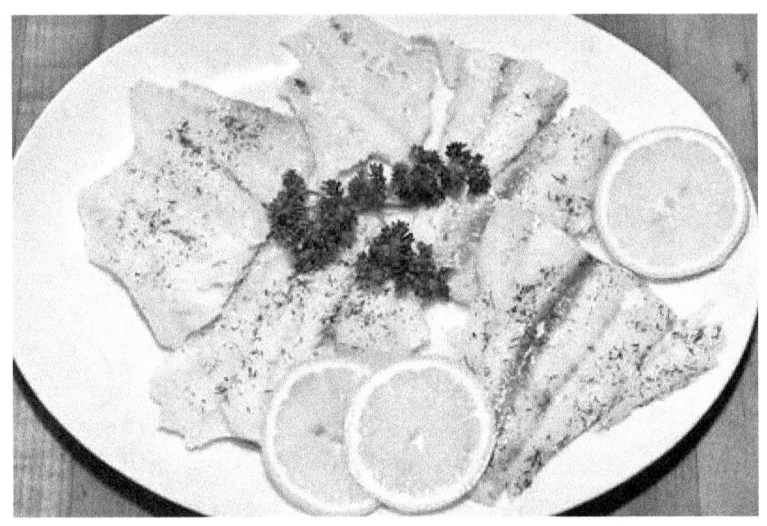

Preparation Time: 10 Minutes

Cooking Time: 12 Minutes

Efforts: Easy

Servings: 4

Nutritional Information per serving:

Calories: 312Kcal, Carbohydrates: 14g, Proteins: 23.1g,

Fat: 18.4g, Sodium: 286mg

Ingredients:

- 1 ½ lb. Cod Fillets
- ¼ cup Parsley leaves, fresh
- 5 cloves of garlic, minced

For lemon juice mixture:
- 2 tbsp. Butter, melted
- 5 tbsp. Lemon Juice, fresh
- 5 tbsp. Extra Virgin Olive Oil

For coating:
- 1/3 cup Almond Flour
- ¾ tsp. Cumin, grounded
- ½ tsp. Black Pepper
- 1 tsp. Coriander, grounded
- ¾ tsp. Salt
- ¾ tsp. Sweet Spanish Paprika

Instructions:
1. Preheat the oven to 400° F.
2. Combine lemon juice, butter, and olive oil in a small-sized mixing bowl. Keep aside. Reserve a bit aside.
3. Combine almond flour, spices, pepper, and salt in another bowl until mixed.
4. Immerse the fish first in the lemon mixture and then in the flour mixture until well coated. Shake off the excess flour.
5. Heat oil in a cast-iron skillet over medium heat, and once the oil starts shimmering, add the fish pieces.
6. Sear them for 3 minutes per side. Set aside the seared fish.
7. Spoon in minced garlic to the remaining lemon mixture and drizzle it over the seared fish.
8. Bake for 9 minutes or until the fish flakes when poked with a fork.
9. Serve it hot.

Tip: Serve along with Greek salad.

GRILLED BEEF & VEGETABLES KABOB

Nut-Free & Dairy-Free

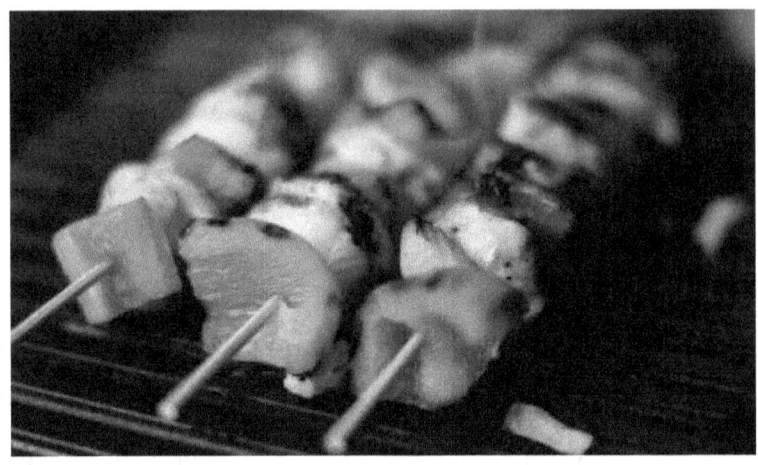

Preparation Time: 10 Minutes + 30 Marinating Time

Cooking Time: 5 Minutes

Efforts: Easy

Servings: 4

Nutritional Information per serving:
Calories: 237Kcal, Carbohydrates: 8.3g, Proteins: 24.8g, Fat: 10.1g, Sodium: 95mg

Ingredients:
- 1 tbsp. Oregano, dried
- ¾ cup Balsamic Vinegar
- ½ tsp. Salt
- ¾ cup Extra-Virgin Olive Oil

- 1 lb. Sirloin Steak, trimmed & chopped into 32 chunks
- 2 Garlic cloves, sliced
- 16 Cherry Tomatoes
- 2 tbsp. Whole Grain Mustard
- 1 tbsp. Rosemary, dried
- ½ tsp. Pepper, grounded
- 16 ×1-inch Red Onion chunks
- 16 Button Mushrooms
- 1 Bell Pepper, cubed into 16 pieces

Instructions:

1. Mix vinegar, pepper, oil, salt, mustard, garlic, oregano, and rosemary in a small mixing bowl.
2. Skewer the meat pieces, bell pepper, mushrooms, onion chunks and tomatoes on eight wooden skewers.
3. Arrange the kebabs on a baking dish and apply the marinade over each of them.
4. Allow it to marinate it for a minimum of ½ hour or a maximum of 8 hours.
5. Preheat the grill to medium-high heat.
6. Remove the excess marinade and take them from the sheet to the grill.
7. Grill them for 7 minutes or until grilled to your desired doneness.
8. Enjoy them hot.

Tip: Serve along with couscous salad.

LENTIL STEW

Under 30 Minutes

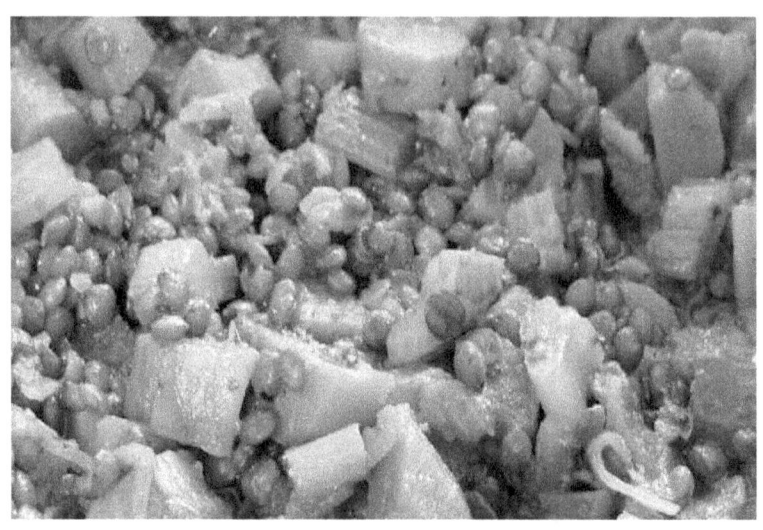

Preparation Time: 10 Minutes

Cooking Time: 20 Minutes

Efforts: Easy

Servings: 4

Nutritional Information per serving:
Calories: 322Kcal, Carbohydrates: 30g, Proteins: 18.8g,

Fat: 5.2g, Sodium: 455mg

Ingredients:
- 2 tbsp. White Wine Vinegar
- 1 tbsp. Olive Oil
- 1 ½ cup Lentils, rinsed
- 2 Garlic cloves, minced

- ½ tsp. Salt
- 2 tbsp. Tomato Paste
- Juice of 1 Lime, large
- 1 ¼ cup Celery, chopped
- ½ cup Red Bell Pepper, chopped finely
- 4 cups Chicken Broth
- 3 Carrots, small & chopped finely
- 5 tbsp. Shallot, finely chopped
- ¾ tsp. Pepper, grounded
- 1 bunch of parsley, fresh & chopped

Instructions:

1. Heat the olive oil in a large-sized pot over medium-high heat.
2. Stir in celery, garlic, carrots, bell pepper, and 2 tbsp. of the shallot.
3. Cook them for 3 minutes or until softened.
4. Spoon in the tomato paste while stirring continuously.
5. Add the lentils, ½ tsp. Pepper and salt along with the broth.
6. Once combined, bring the stew mixture to a boil.
7. Reduce heat. Allow it to simmer for 38 minutes while keeping it covered.
8. Transfer the stew to a serving bowl and serve it hot.

Tip: Serve it along with salsa verde.

GARDEN PASTA SALAD

Under 30 Minutes

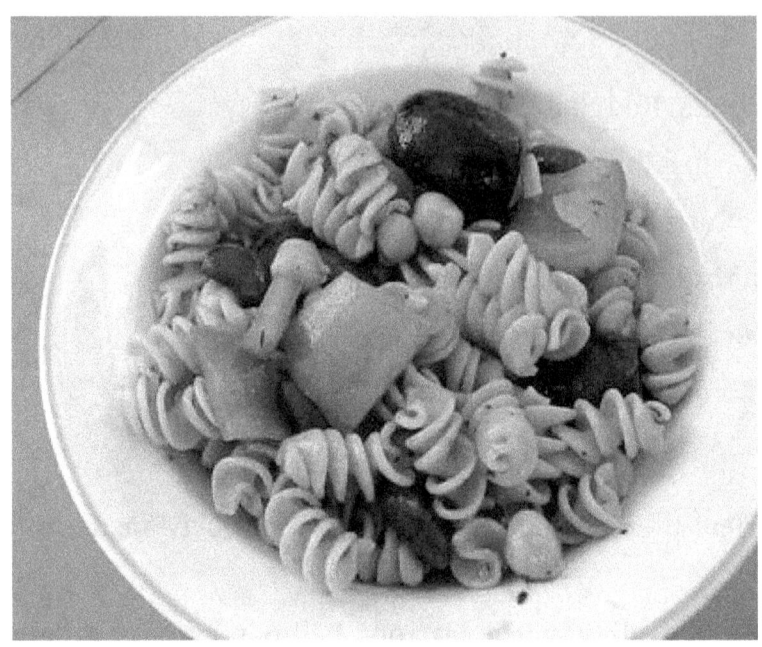

Preparation Time: 10 Minutes

Cooking Time: 10 Minutes

Efforts: Easy

Servings: 8

Nutritional Information per serving:

Calories: 241Kcal, Carbohydrates: 25g, Proteins: 18.1g,

Fat: 5.3g, Sodium: 284mg

Ingredients:
- 1 tsp. Red Pepper Flakes
- 1 cup Chickpeas, cooked
- 6 cups whole-wheat Pasta, cooked
- ¾ cup Red Bell Pepper, chopped
- 4 oz. Black Olives, sliced & drained
- ¾ cup Onion, chopped finely
- ¾ cup Zucchini, sliced
- ¼ cup Parsley, fresh & chopped
- ½ cup Lemon Juice
- Salt, as needed
- ½ cup Parmesan Cheese, low-fat & shredded

Instructions:
1. Place all the ingredients excluding lemon juice and parsley in a large mixing bowl. Toss well.
2. Pour the lemon juice over the salad and garnish it with the parsley leaves.
3. Serve and enjoy.

Tip: The salad tastes the best when served chill.

POTATO SOUP

Nut-Free

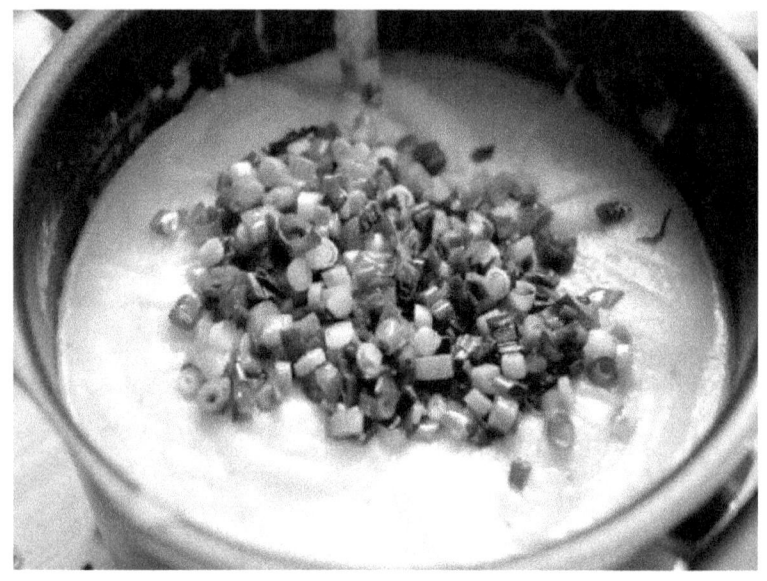

Preparation Time: 5 Minutes

Cooking Time: 25 Minutes

Efforts: Easy

Servings: 6

Nutritional Information per serving:

Calories: 565Kcal, Carbohydrates: 18g, Proteins: 6g,

Fat: 4.1g, Sodium: 302mg

Ingredients:

- 1 tbsp. Olive Oil
- 5 Potatoes, boiled with their skin & diced
- 2 handful of Chives, fresh & chopped
- 1 Onion, medium & chopped finely
- 1 Garlic clove, crushed
- 1 Onion, medium & diced finely
- 2 ½ cup Vegetable Stock
- A dollop of Sour Cream

Instructions:

1. Cook the onion and garlic in a large pot over medium-high heat.
2. Once softened, stir in the potatoes and then pour the stock to it.
3. Bring the soup to a boil and allow it to simmer for 12 minutes.
4. Set it aside for a few minutes to cool. Transfer the potato mixture to a high-speed blender and blend for a minute until smooth.
5. Bring the soup back to the pot and heat it through.
6. Transfer to a bowl and top it with the chives and sour cream.
7. Serve it hot.

Tip: You can add water if it seems too thickened.

BLACK BEAN SOUP

Nut - Free

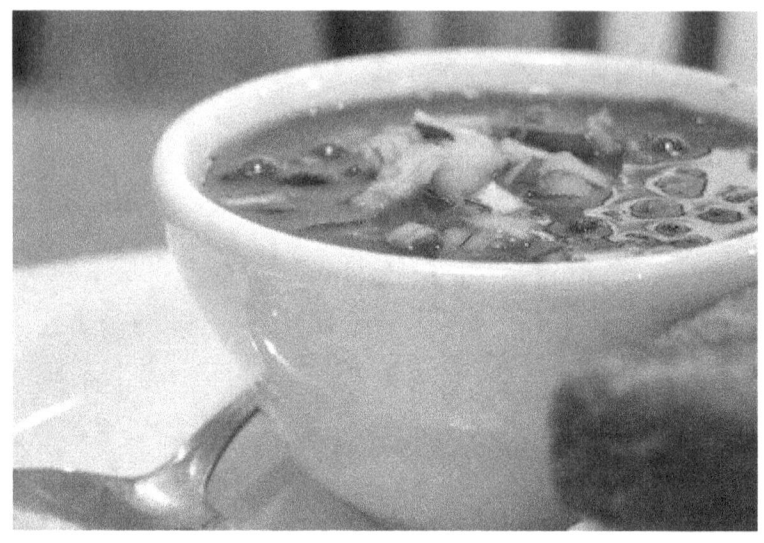

Preparation Time: 5 Minutes

Cooking Time: 25 Minutes

Efforts: Easy

Servings: 6

Nutritional Information per serving:

Calories: 296Kcal, Carbohydrates: 23g, Proteins: 19g,

Fat: 9g, Sodium: 302mg

Ingredients:
- 1 Onion, diced
- 6 tbsp. Parmesan, grated
- 1 tbsp. Tomato Paste
- 1 tbsp. Extra Virgin Olive Oil
- 1 cob of Corn, kernels removed

- 2 Carrots, diced finely
- 6 tsp. Yogurt
- 1 tsp. Thyme, fresh & chopped
- 1 tbsp. Tamari
- 1 clove of garlic, crushed
- 1 tbsp. Extra Virgin Olive Oil
- 1 Red Bell Pepper, diced finely
- 1 tsp. Cumin, grounded
- 1 cup Black Beans, soaked overnight
- 14 oz. Sweet potato, diced
- 1 tbsp. Coriander, fresh & chopped finely

Instructions:

1. Soak the chickpeas, add the yogurt to the water and stir. Set it aside.
2. Sspoon in oil to a large pot and add the onion to it.
3. Sauté them for 3 minutes or until softened. Spoon in thyme, garlic, coriander, and cumin.
4. Sauté for another 3 minutes and add all the remaining ingredients into it, excluding the tamari, coriander, and parmesan.
5. Cover the pot and cook for 3 hours while checking it now and then until everything comes together.
6. Add the tamari. Serve it with yogurt, coriander, and parmesan.
7. Serve it hot.

Tip: If preferred, you can spoon in the chipotle sauce to it for more spiciness.

SHRIMP & AVOCADO SALAD

Keto & Under 30 Minutes

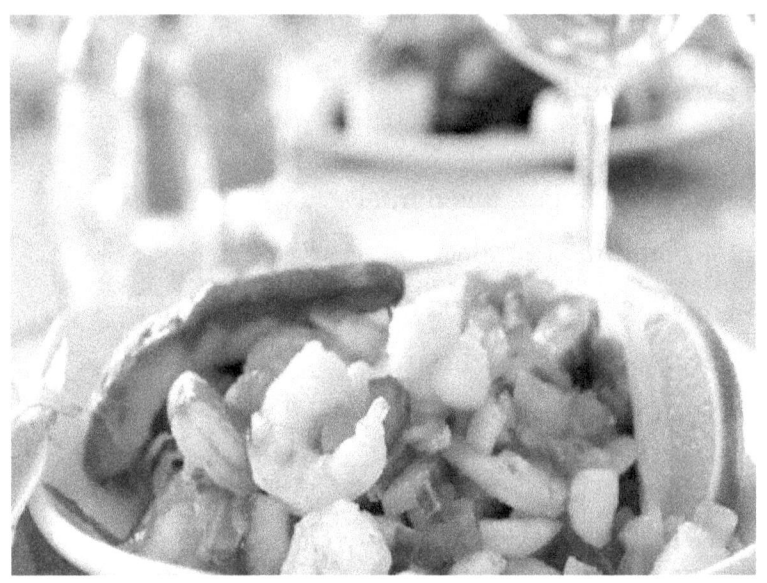

Preparation Time: 20 Minutes

Cooking Time: 0 Minutes

Efforts: Easy

Servings: 4

Nutritional Information per serving:
Calories: 197Kcal, Carbohydrates: 4g, Proteins: 25g,
Fat: 8g, Sodium: 330mg

Ingredients:
- Juice of 2 Limes
- 1 tbsp. Cilantro, chopped
- ¼ cup Red Onion, chopped
- 1 Avocado, medium & diced
- 1 tsp. Olive Oil
- 1 Jalapeno, deseeded & diced finely
- Salt & pepper, as needed
- 1 Tomato, medium & diced
- 1 lb. Jumbo Prawns, cooked & chopped

Instructions:

1. Mix red onion, pepper, lime juice, salt, and olive oil in a medium-sized mixing bowl. Keep it aside for 5 minutes for the flavors to meld.
2. Place the shrimp, jalapeno, avocado, and jalapeno in another bowl.
3. Combine everything until everything comes together. Add cilantro, salt, and pepper. Stir.
4. Serve and enjoy.

Tip: Serve it along with tostada for a complete meal.

DINNER

CREAM OF ASPARAGUS SOUP

Keto & Nut-free

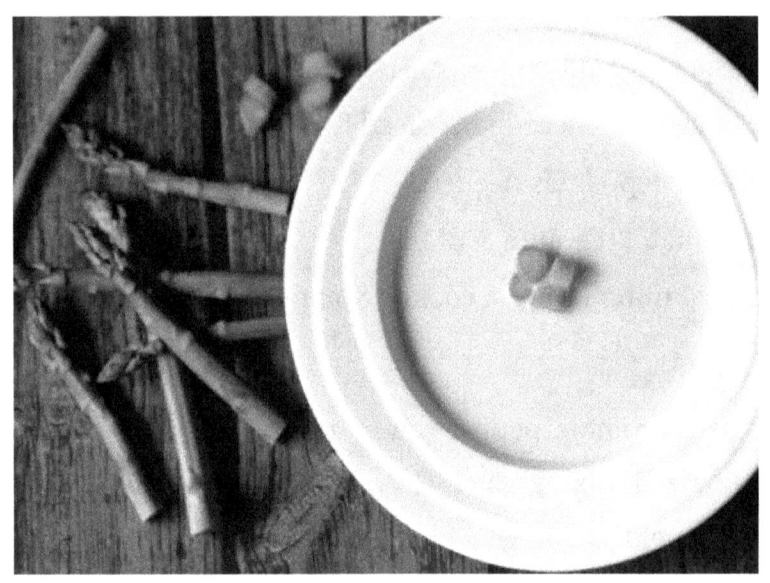

Preparation Time: 5 Minutes

Cooking Time: 25 Minutes

Efforts: Easy

Servings: 6

Nutritional Information per serving:
Calories: 81Kcal, Carbohydrates: 6g, Proteins: 6g, Fat: 3g, Sodium: 576mg

Ingredients:

- 2 lb. Asparagus
- 2 tbsp. Low-fat Sour Cream
- 1 tbsp. Butter, unsalted
- 6 cups Chicken broth
- Salt & pepper, as needed
- 1 Onion, medium & chopped

Instructions:

1. Spoon butter into a heated pot over medium-high heat.
2. Stir in onion and saute for 2 minutes or until softened.
3. After that, slice the asparagus into two and stir into the pot along with the chicken broth.
4. Allow it to boil and reduce the heat.
5. Cook for 18 minutes or until the asparagus is tender.
6. Take off the pot from the heat and spoon in sour cream. Keep it aside to cool.
7. Once cooled, transfer to a high-speed blender and puree it until smooth.
8. Serve and enjoy.

Tip: You can serve it with a simple green salad. If desired, you can add crumbled bacon or parmesan cheese to it.

ADOBO CHICKEN

Keto, Diary-Free & Nut-Free

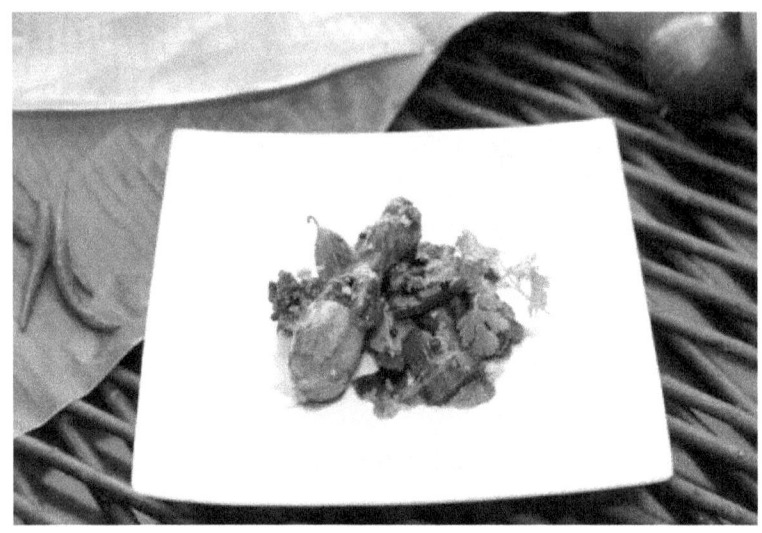

Preparation Time: 10 Minutes

Cooking Time: 60 Minutes

Efforts: Easy

Servings: 4

Nutritional Information per serving:
Calories: 175Kcal, Carbohydrates: 4.5g, Proteins: 27g,

Fat: 4.5g, Sodium: 620mg

Ingredients:

- 4 Bay Leaves
- 8 Chicken Drumsticks, skinless & on the bone
- 6 Peppercorns, grounded
- 1/3 cup Soy Sauce, low-sodium
- 1/3 cup Apple Cider Vinegar
- 1 head of garlic, small & crushed

Instructions:

1. Season the chicken drumsticks with soy sauce, pepper, vinegar, and garlic in a mixing bowl. Set it aside for 1 hour or overnight.
2. Heat a deep non-stick skillet on medium-low heat and place the marinated chicken, bay leaves, and ½ cup water in it.
3. Cook the meat for 40 minutes or until it becomes tender while keeping it covered.
4. Open the lid and continue cooking for another 15 minutes while the liquid gets absorbed.
5. Remove the bay leaves and serve it hot.

Tip: To spice up, you can add one jalapeno to it.

CAULIFLOWER SOUP

Keto & Under 30 Minutes

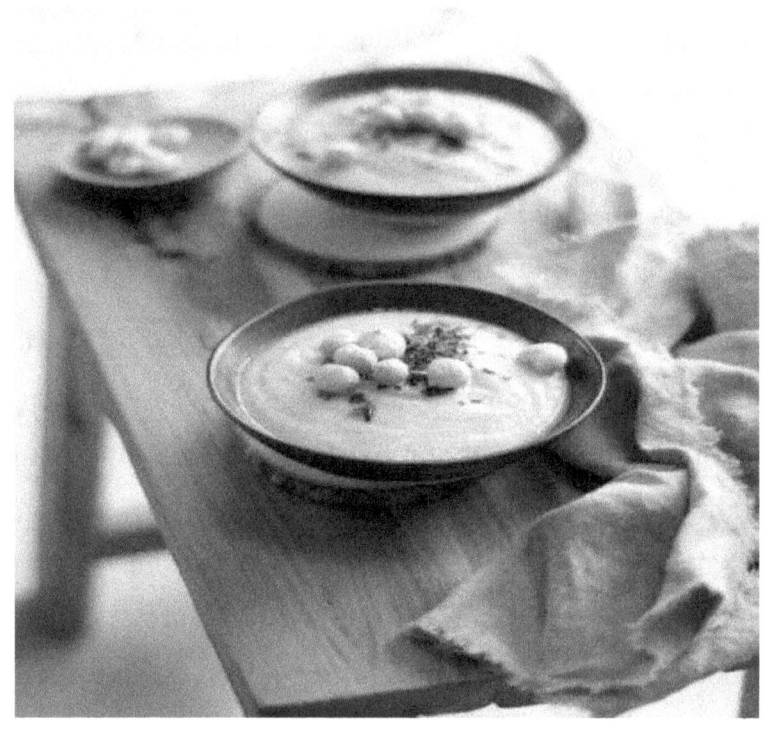

Preparation Time: 5 Minutes

Cooking Time: 15 Minutes

Efforts: Easy

Servings: 4

Nutritional Information per serving:

Calories: 196Kcal, Carbohydrates: 7g, Proteins: 4g,

Fat: 16g, Sodium: 314mg

Ingredients:
- 1 Cauliflower head, torn into florets
- ¾ of 1 Onion, sliced
- ¼ tsp. Nutmeg, grounded
- 2 Garlic cloves
- ½ tsp. Thyme
- ½ cup Heavy Cream
- ½ tsp. Black Pepper
- 2 cups Water
- 1 Chicken Stock Cube
- Salt, as needed
- 1 tsp. Olive Oil

Instructions:
1. Heat the oil in a heavy-bottomed saucepan over medium heat.
2. Stir in the onions and saute for 3 minutes or until softened.
3. Add the cauliflower and raise the heat to medium-high.
4. Continue cooking until it becomes slightly browned and roasted.
5. Spoon in the garlic, pepper, thyme, nutmeg, and stock cube to it. Stir well.
6. Pour the water and deglaze it so that the browned bits sticking to the bottom comes up.
7. Allow it to a simmer and cook for 13 minutes on low heat until the cauliflower becomes tender. Set it aside to cool.
8. Once cooled, transfer to a high-speed blender and blend for 2 minutes or until you get a smooth mixture.
9. Strain the mixture Pour the soup back to the saucepan and heat it through.
10. Spoon in the heavy cream and give everything a mix.
11. Serve it hot.

Tip: If you prefer to make it cheesy, you can add ¼ cup of your favorite cheese to it.

BUTTER CHICKEN

Keto & Nut-Free

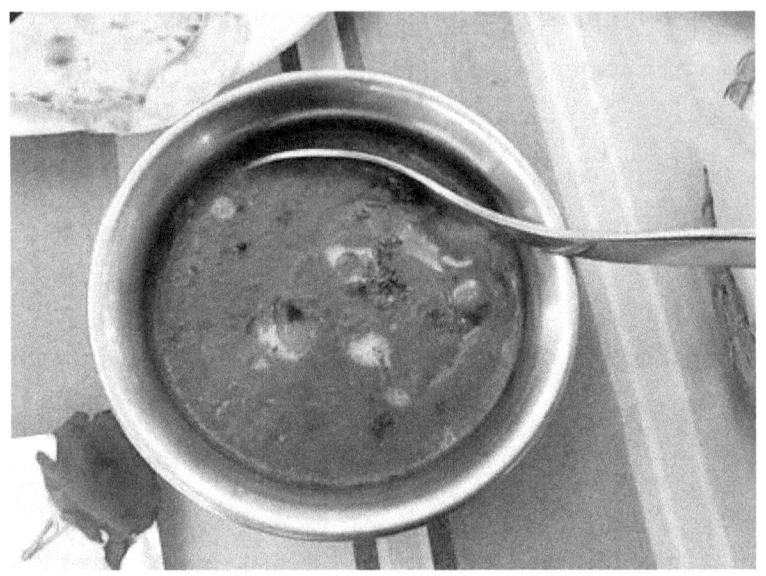

Preparation Time: 10 Minutes

Cooking Time: 30 Minutes

Efforts: Easy

Servings: 4

Nutritional Information per serving:
Calories: 385Kcal, Carbohydrates: 6g, Proteins: 26.5g, Fat: 26.75g, Sodium: 433mg

Ingredients:
- ½ tsp. Cinnamon, grounded
- 1 lb. Chicken Breast, chopped into bite-size chunks
- ¾ tsp. Chili Powder

- 2 tbsp. Butter
- 1 tsp. Pink Himalayan Salt
- 1 ½ tbsp. Tomato Paste
- 1 tsp. Ginger, grounded
- 2 Garlic cloves
- 1 ½ tsp. Turmeric Powder
- ¼ of 1 Onion, medium & diced
- 1 cup Heavy Cream

Instructions:

1. Marinate the chicken pieces with turmeric, cinnamon, ginger, chili powder, and salt. Coat thoroughly and keep it aside.
2. Melt butter in a medium skillet over medium heat.
3. Add the onion and garlic. Saute for 2 minutes or until aromatic.
4. Raise the heat to medium-high heat and stir in the chicken.
5. Continue cooking for another 5 minutes or until the chicken is cooked.
6. Pour the cream and tomato paste to it. Stir well and lower the heat to medium-low.
7. Cook for 7 minutes while keeping it covered. Open the lid and cook for further 2 minutes or until the sauce has thickened.
8. Serve it hot.

Tip: Serve it with cauliflower rice.

THAI TOFU CURRY

Keto & Under 30 Minutes

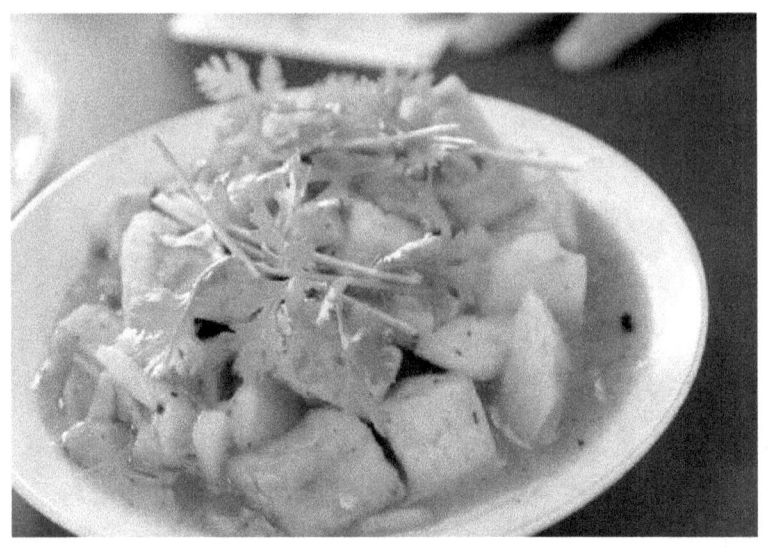

Preparation Time: 10 Minutes

Cooking Time: 15 Minutes

Efforts: Easy

Servings: 4

Nutritional Information per serving:
Calories: 318Kcal, Carbohydrates: 7g, Proteins: 12g,

Fat: 27.1g, Sodium: 433mg

Ingredients:
- 1 Garlic clove
- 1 packet of Tofu, cubed
- ¼ cup Soy Sauce
- 2 Bell Peppers, sliced into strips

- 1 Lemon Grass Stalks
- 2 tbsp. Coconut Oil
- 1-inch Ginger, minced
- 1 tbsp. Tomato Paste
- 1 tbsp. Butter
- 15 oz. Coconut Milk
- 1 tsp. Thai Curry Paste
- 2 tsp. Chili Flakes

Instructions:

1. Heat a large-sized saucepan over medium heat and spoon in the oil to it.
2. Add the garlic and ginger. Saute until aromatic.
3. Stir in bell pepper and lemongrass stalks. Cook for 25 seconds and pour coconut milk and chili flakes to it.
4. Mix well and add soy sauce, tomato paste, curry paste, and butter to it. Stir for a minute.
5. Spoon in the tofu pieces and cook for 8 minutes or until the sauce is thickened.
6. Remove the pan from the heat Transfer to a bowl and serve it hot.

Tip: Top it with coriander and green onions.

CABBAGE SLAW

Under 30 Minutes & Less than 5 Ingredients

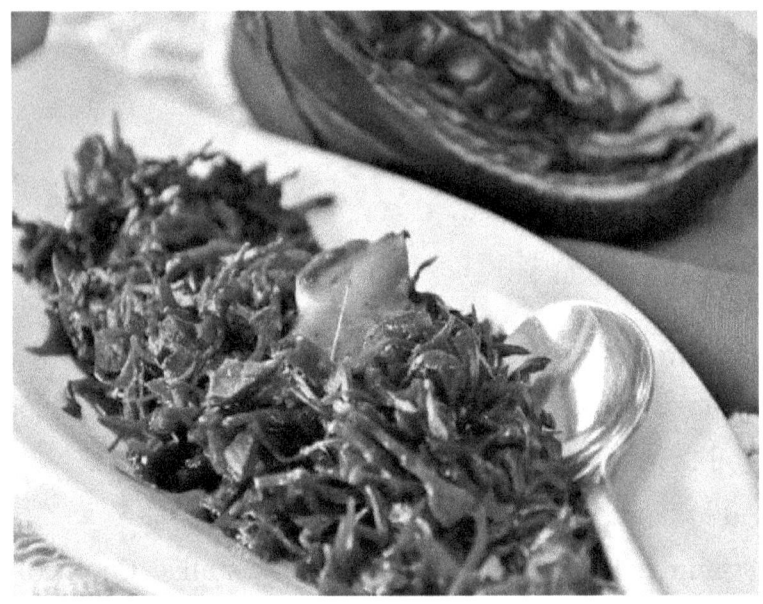

Preparation Time: 15 Minutes

Cooking Time: 0 Minutes

Efforts: Easy

Servings: 4

Nutritional Information per serving:
Calories: 88Kcal, Carbohydrates: 5g, Proteins: 1g,

Fat: 7g, Sodium: 255mg

Ingredients:

- ¼ tsp. Salt
- ½ of 1 small Purple Cabbage head
- 5 tsp. Apple Cider Vinegar
- ½ of 1 Red Bell Pepper
- 2 tbsp. Extra Virgin Olive Oil
- ¼ of 1 Red Onion, small
- Black Pepper, as needed

Instructions:

1. Place all the ingredients in the large mixing bowl and mix well.
2. Set it aside for 15 minutes before serving.

Tip: Top it with coriander and green onions.

FIVE-SPICE CHICKEN DRUMSTICKS

Diary-Free

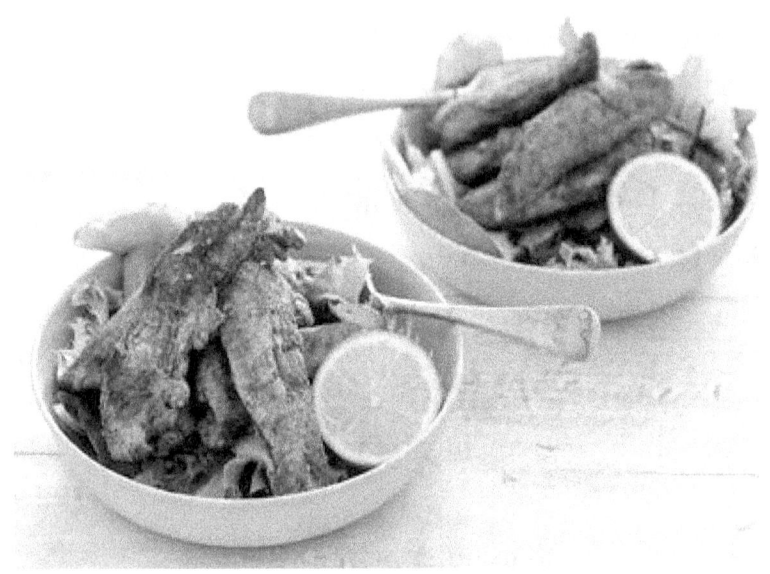

Preparation Time: 5 Minutes

Cooking Time: 30 Minutes

Efforts: Easy

Servings: 2

Nutritional Information per serving:
Calories: 88Kcal, Carbohydrates: 5g, Proteins: 1g,

Fat: 7g, Sodium: 255mg

Ingredients:
- 6 Chicken Drumsticks
- 2 tbsp. Olive Oil
- 1 Green Onion, sliced
- 3 tbsp. Soy Sauce
- Cilantro, fresh & chopped
- 2 tsp. Chinese Five Spice Powder
- Salt & pepper, as needed

Instructions:
1. Combine soy sauce, five-spice powder, oil, and salt in a large mixing bowl.
2. Place the chicken thighs and coat it thoroughly with the seasonings.
3. Keep it in the refrigerator for at least half an hour or a few hours, if possible.
4. Preheat it for 400°F.
5. Arrange the drumsticks on a greased baking sheet.
6. Roast for 25 minutes or until the thermometer shows 165°C.
7. Garnish it with coriander and spring onions.

Tip: You can serve it along with cabbage stir fry for a complete meal.

TOMATO GAZPACHO

Less than 30 Minutes

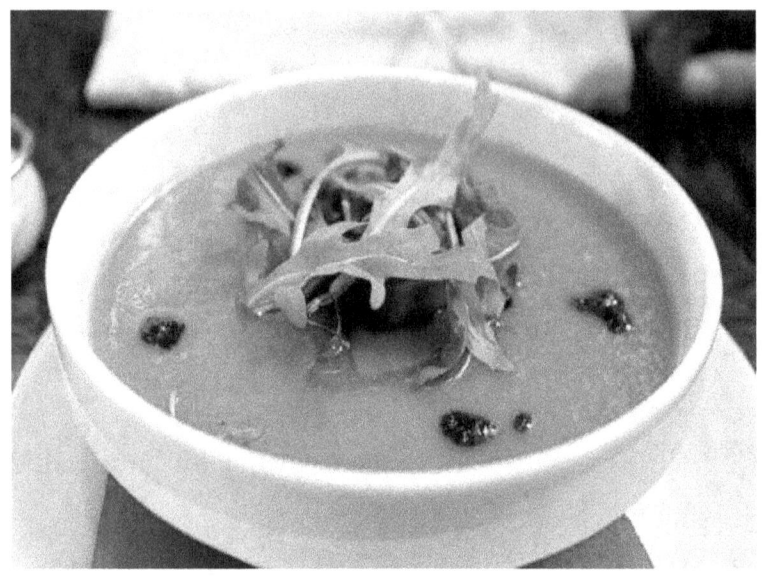

Preparation Time: 15 Minutes

Cooking Time: 0 Minutes

Efforts: Easy

Servings: 2

Nutritional Information per serving:
Calories: 82.1Kcal, Carbohydrates: 7g, Proteins: 1.7g,

Fat: 5.1g, Sodium: 13mg

Ingredients:

- ¼ of 1 Red Bell Pepper
- 2 tbsp. Red onion, chopped
- ½ of 1 Cucumber, medium, peeled & seeded
- 2 tsp. Extra Virgin Olive Oil
- 1 clove of Garlic
- 2 Tomatoes, large
- Salt & pepper, as needed
- 1 tsp. Red Wine Vinegar

Instructions:

1. Place tomatoes, garlic, cucumber, salt, vinegar, garlic, and salt in a high-speed blender.
2. Blend for a minute or until it becomes smooth.
3. Place it in the refrigerator for at least half an hour.
4. Transfer the soup to the serving bowl and spoon one teaspoon of olive oil over it.
5. Top it with red onion, salt, and pepper.
6. Serve it hot.

Tip: Serve it along with grilled shrimp.

CONCLUSION

Diabetic foods are the perfect solution to enjoy healthy foods at home every day. Recipes prepared according to these guidelines take care of not only your health but also your cravings to enjoy delicious foods. They greatly assist in keeping your weight under check.

This book aims at educating readers about the benefit of switching to a healthy diabetic lifestyle without compromising on taste. Dedicated efforts have been made in the book to provide its readers with healthy recipes that they can prepare at home anytime they want and enjoy them guilt-free.

We thank you all for giving their precious time to read this book. We sincerely hope that the recipes covered in the book will inspire its readers to start eating healthy foods. Start your journey by making your first diabetic-friendly recipe from this book, and continue enjoying the savory treats.

Thank you all again; good luck!

© Copyright by Karen Berenice Harper 2020 - All rights reserved.

The content contained within this book may not be reproduced, duplicated or transmitted without direct written permission from the author or the publisher.

Under no circumstances will any blame or legal responsibility be held against the publisher, or author, for any damages, reparation, or monetary loss due to the information contained within this book. Either directly or indirectly. You are responsible for your own choices, actions, and results.

Legal Notice:

This book is copyright protected. This book is only for personal use. You cannot amend, distribute, sell, use, quote or paraphrase any part, or the content within this book, without the consent of the author or publisher.

Disclaimer Notice:

Please note the information contained within this document is for educational and entertainment purposes only. All effort has been executed to present accurate, up to date, and reliable, complete information. No warranties of any kind are declared or implied. Readers acknowledge that the author is not engaging in the rendering of legal, financial, medical or professional advice. The content within this book has been derived from various sources. Please consult a licensed professional before attempting any techniques outlined in this book.

By reading this document, the reader agrees that under no circumstances is the author responsible for any losses, direct or indirect, which are incurred as a result of the use of the information contained within this document, including, but not limited to, — errors, omissions, or inaccuracies.

www.ingramcontent.com/pod-product-compliance
Lightning Source LLC
Chambersburg PA
CBHW052341220526
45465CB00003BA/906